7887

Pressure garments

A manual on their design and fabrication

Joanne Pratt MSc, Dip COT, OTR
Gill West Dip COT, SROT

Illustrated by Brian Withinshaw

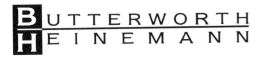
BUTTERWORTH
HEINEMANN

Butterworth-Heinemann Ltd
Linacre House, Jordan Hill, Oxford OX2 8DP

℟ A member of the Reed Elsevier plc group

OXFORD   LONDON   BOSTON
MUNICH   NEW DELHI   SINGAPORE   SYDNEY
TOKYO   TORONTO   WELLINGTON

First edition 1995

© Butterworth-Heinemann Ltd 1995

The authors are not responsible for injuries arising out of use or misuse
of these materials. This includes but is not limited to: failure to follow
instructions; failure to heed any cautions noted in the text, diagrams or charts;
use of pressure therapy without medical guidance. It is presumed that the user
of these materials has an awareness of the limitations which might contraindicate
the use of pressure therapy and will consult medical personnel where appropriate.
The user should read the text, particularly the first two chapters, before attempting
to make garments

British Library Cataloguing in Publication Data
Pratt, Joanne
  Pressure Garments: A Manual on Their Design
  and Fabrication
  I. Title II. West, Gill III. Withinshaw,
  Brian
  615.822
ISBN 0 7506 2064 1

Library of Congress Cataloguing in Publication Data
Pratt, Joanne.
  Pressure garments: a manual on their design and fabrication/
  Joanne Pratt, Gill West; illustrated by Brain Withinshaw. — 1st ed.
  p. cm.
  Includes bibliographical references and index.
  ISBN 0 7506 2064 1
  1. Pressure suits — Therapeutic use. I. West, Gill. II. Title.
  RM827. P73   1994
  681'.761   dc20

94–33550
CIP

Typeset by TecSet Ltd, Wallington, Surrey
Printed in Great Britain The Bath Press, Avon

Contents

About the authors

Joanne Pratt attended the Derby School of Occupational Therapy in England, qualifying in 1982. She first encountered pressure therapy as a student on an elective placement in Hong Kong, and then at Withington Hospital, Manchester, England. Her MSc thesis investigated the outcome of pressure therapy on hypertrophic scarring using an ultrasound scanner to measure dermal thickness in patients seven years post-discharge. Joanne has had diverse work experience as a clinician in physical and mental dysfunction in several countries. She is currently employed as a lecturer in the Division of Occupational Therapy, Glasgow Caledonian University, Scotland.

Gill West qualified in 1982 from the Dorset House School of Occupational Therapy, Oxford, England. She first encountered pressure therapy while working at the Regional Burns and Plastic Surgery Unit, Withington Hospital, Manchester, England. Gill has had varied clinical experience in physical dysfunction, including six years in the rehabilitation of people with upper limb amputations. She has worked in Britain and Canada. She is currently employed as a Senior I occupational therapist in orthopaedics and rheumatology at Arrowe Park Hospital, Merseyside, England.

Acknowledgements

The assistance of a number of people was helpful in the preparation of this manual and is acknowledged with gratitude.

Joyce Smith, Technical Instructor, taught and encouraged both authors to develop the art and skill necessary to make pressure garments. She was generous with her time, knowledge and sense of humour, despite all!

The Occupational Therapy Department at Withington Hospital, Manchester, allowed the use of their information sheets for this project.

We would like to thank all our former and present patients for allowing us to learn more about pressure therapy and its efficacy.

Finally, we gratefully acknowledge the support and encouragement of our families.

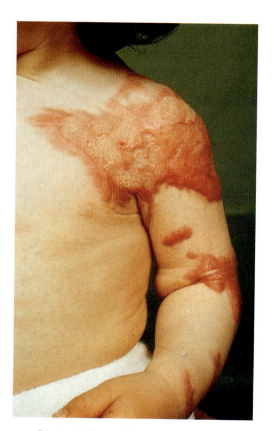 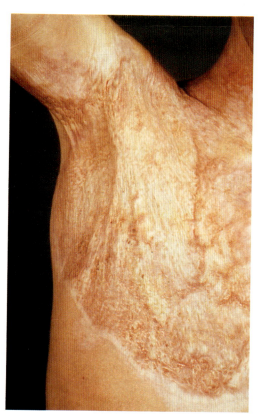

Plate 1 The red, raised and rigid appearance of hypertrophic scars in a child (left) and an adult (right).

1

Pressure therapy: history and rationale

A burn injury can be both a physically and emotionally traumatic experience. Children under the age of 5 years represent the group most at risk for this type of injury, largely caused by scalds. Fortunately for the majority of burned patients their wounds heal, so that eventually there is little to distinguish the site of injury from the surrounding skin. However, this is not so for all patients. A significant number of them will develop scars at the original site of injury. Wounds caused by injuries other than by burn usually develop scars which resolve in a matter of months. Burn scars can become red and raised with a lumpy appearance and because of their size are referred to as *hypertrophic* scars. They can remain active, i.e. red, raised and itchy, for a much longer period of time than other scars (see Plate 1). They have been observed to persist for 12 months in Caucasian adults, 24 months in Caucasian children, and occasionally for more than 48 months in Black and Oriental peoples.

The box below highlights the main problems caused by hypertrophic scars. We will consider each of them more closely.

> **Problems caused by hypertrophic scars**
> - **Itchiness**
> - **Disfigurement**
> - **Contractures**

Itchiness

The increased blood supply which causes the red appearance of the hypertrophic scar can also cause the sensation of itchiness (pruritus) which can increase to the point of discomfort for some patients.

Disfigurement

Hypertrophic scars are red and unsightly, drawing attention to an injury. If the scar site is on a very noticeable area like the face, it can be disfiguring, altering the patient's appearance considerably. This change in appearance is often permanent, and psychological adjustment problems can follow and will need attention.

Contractures

Where a scar is large enough to cover a joint it can decrease the range of movement in that joint because scars tighten as they heal. If the scar tissue is not kept supple through massage and regular movement of the joint, then a contracture can develop.

A patient can experience any one or all of these problems. Their ability to carry out their daily activities, including those of personal care, work and leisure interests, will be compromised.

The aim of this manual is to describe in practical detail one method used to manage hypertrophic scarring, i.e. elasticated garments, hereafter referred to as pressure garments. This treatment developed following early observations that pressure, from bandages or splints for example, appeared to result in flatter scars.

In order to describe how pressure garments are designed and fabricated we have organized this manual as follows:

> **Manual content**
> - **Rationale of pressure therapy**
> - **Indications for pressure therapy**
> - **Measurement, sewing and design advice**
> - **Individual garment instructions**

It is hoped that this information will be especially useful to those practitioners who are hoping to develop a pressure therapy service and to those who wish to develop greater understanding of the mechanics and challenges of applying pressure to human tissue.

It is anticipated that a number of terms used in the text may be new to readers. Highlight boxes will be used to define keywords, with diagrams to support the text.

This chapter continues with a consideration of skin structure, burn wound healing and a review of the methods used to manage hypertrophic scarring.

Normal skin structure

Keywords

Epidermis. The outermost or visible part of skin, which is composed of three *strata* or layers, the *stratum basale, stratum spinosum* and *stratum granulosum*

Dermis. That layer of skin which lies just beneath the epidermis

Collagen. A protein which occurs in 11 different forms in the body as a major constituent of connective tissue, i.e. dermis, bones, muscles, cartilage, blood vessels

Desmosomes. Microscopic connections between those cells in the stratum basale of the dermis and those immediately above them in the stratum spinosum

Squamous. The top layer of dead cells which are shed from skin during normal daily hygiene activities.

Human skin is comprised of two distinct layers, the epidermis and the dermis. It serves as the border between the body's internal and external environments and, as such, assists in maintenance of the internal state – temperature control, electrolyte balance, etc. It also provides a first line of defence or a barrier against infection. Both the structure and the functions of skin can be seriously disrupted by burn injury.

The epidermis is outermost and has been described as a many-layered pavement of epithelial cells. The epidermis is maintained by a process in which cells bud off in the lowest layer, the *stratum basale*, which is the only point in the epidermis at which cell division occurs. The cells then travel upwards through the epidermis, during which they undergo a progression of differentiation. Cells first become cuboidal, linked to other cells by desmosomes in the *stratum spinosum*. On travelling to the upper limits of the *stratum granulosum* they begin to lose their nuclei and become filled with dark-staining lipid granules. Above the *stratum granulosum* the cells degenerate into the metabolically inactive squamous cells which humans gradually shed from the skin surface. The epidermis has no blood supply but relies on the diffusion of nutrients from the vessels present in the upper layer of the dermis.

The dermis is divided into a superficial papillary layer and a deeper reticular layer which borders the subcutaneous fat. Collagen, the structural component of the dermis, is a generic term for 11 types of molecule formed by fibrous proteins. It provides the structure in skin, bone and tendon. Collagen's distinguishing characteristic is its ability to adhere both side to side and end to end. This allows it to form bundles. Type I collagen forms the core of these bundles while types III and V limit the size of bundles from their position on the periphery. While collagen occurs primarily in bundles, individual filaments can also be seen running parallel to the skin surface throughout the interstitial space. The dermis also contains mast cells which release histamines when damaged. These cells are thought to have a significant role in scar remodelling.

Wound healing

Keywords

Platelets. Cells found in blood which are important in clotting

Neutrophils. A type of white blood cell

Macrophages. Cells formed by the body to fight infection

Phenotype. A template from which variations derive as needed

Angiogenesis. The formation of new blood vessels

Homeostasis. A condition of physiological stability within the body's internal environment

Fibroplasia. Production of fibroblast cells, essential for the construction of a wound matrix

Wound healing is thought to have three phases, but these should not be viewed as sequential stages as there may be considerable overlap:

Three phases of wound healing

- **Inflammation**
- **Granulation formation**
- **Matrix formation and remodelling**

Inflammation phase

During the early inflammatory phase, platelets in the wound site are activated by the disruption to blood vessels from the injury. They trigger blood coagulation, thereby influencing blood homeostasis in addition to releasing substances which promote cell migration to the area of injury. Neutrophils and monocytes are among those which infiltrate the area first; the latter then alter phenotype to become macrophages. Together neutrophils and macrophages serve to clear the site of debris. Macrophages are thought to perform several roles during wound repair, but function mainly in the inflammatory phase to help prepare the area for the formation of granulation tissue.

Granulation formation

Granulation tissue (Figure 1.1) can be thought of as the infill in a wound area. It is comprised of macrophages, fibroblasts and neovasculature which work in conjunction to (a) deposit a matrix which both

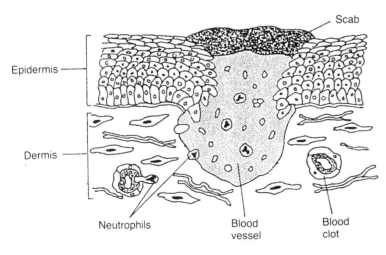

Figure 1.1 **Granulation tissue**

supports and promotes the growth of further granulations, and (b) stimulate wound contraction. Fibroblasts deposit fibronectin in a loose extracellular matrix when they migrate into the wound site. This matrix can then be used for movement of other cells across the wound surface. This process of fibroplasia contributes to the second function of granulation tissue, i.e. wound contraction, by the activation of myofibroblasts which align along the lines of contraction and are thus credited with wound closure. The presence of this matrix also provides a base from which collagen production can occur.

Re-epithelialization (Figure 1.2) also takes place during the granulation phase. There is a rapid increase in the number of epithelial cells from the remaining sources which migrate across the wound infill, gradually re-forming it. This process alters if the basal membrane has remained intact, as alteration of the hemidesmosomes is needed and performed to allow epithelial mobility. Once the migrating cells return to phenotype, these attachments to the basal membrane are re-established.

Angiogenesis occurs simultaneously with re-epithelialization when capillary buds sprout from blood vessels which lie adjacent to the wound site. Low oxygen tension, the presence of lactic acid and/or macrophages may all play a part in stimulating angiogenesis.

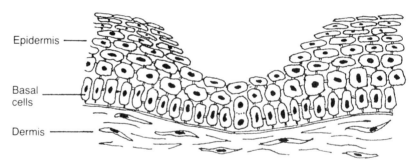

Epidermis

Basal cells

Dermis

Figure 1.2 **Epithelialization**

Matrix formation and remodelling

The loose extracellular matrix formed by fibrin, fibronectin and new collagen is replaced by a slow accumulation of type I collagen in bundles, which provides the scar with strength. The presence of growth factors modulates fibroblast production of both fibronectin and collagen.

During the remodelling phase, the matrix matures such that collagen bundles grow in both size and strength to replace fibronectin and hyaluronic acid which disappear. Proteoglycans are also deposited and add to the resilience of the tissue. New basement membrane which anchors the epithelium to the interstitium matures last. Its reformation starts early in the wound repair process and concludes when anchoring strands, formed from type VII collagen fibrils, re-establish the epidermal–neodermal association.

Burn wound healing

> **Keywords**
>
> **Necrosis.** Tissue death
>
> **Debridement.** Removal of necrotic tissue by several means, e.g. baths, manual removal
>
> **Excision.** Surgical removal of necrotic tissue
>
> **Escharotomy.** Surgical incision through burned tissue, especially in the case of circumferential burns
>
> **Graft.** Cover for a burn site from a donor area, usually from the patient themselves. The split thickness skin graft (STSG) is mainly used while the mesh graft is used to cover large areas

Burn wound healing differs from this in a number of ways. First, and most striking, is the initial response to trauma. Burn injury sites do not bleed. The blood flow in the veins and arteries that remain following the burn is blocked. Capillaries lose their integrity, and become so permeable that cell membranes may disappear in extreme cases. This is particularly marked in injuries greater than total burn surface area (TBSA) 30% (Figure 1.3).

'Depth' of wound is a term which merits consideration because of its profound implications for wound healing. Every increase in burn depth correspondingly decreases the likelihood of spontaneous recovery. This situation arises because there are fewer sources of epithelium, critical to the generation of new cells, as a wound deepens. Depth is classified as being of (a) superficial partial thickness, (b) (deep) partial thickness, or (c) full thickness. 'Mixed depth' and 'deep dermal' are also used as terms to describe wound severity.

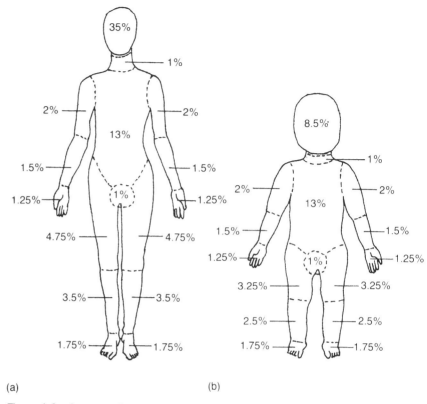

Figure 1.3 **A comparison of (a) adult and (b) infant (1 year old) body surface area calculations (by percentage): anterior views**

Keywords

First-degree burn. Involves only the epidermis. Skin functions remain intact

Second-degree burn. Involves the epidermis and possibly parts of the dermis. Blistering occurs.

Partial thickness burns. First- and second-degree burns, collectively

Third-degree burn. Destroys the epidermis, dermis, and epidermal derivatives like sweat glands and hair follicles. These are also known as *full thickness burns*

In the case of a superficial injury, i.e. involving the epidermis and/or the superficial papillary dermis, new skin cover will arise from the remaining epithelial cells which border the wound, the hair follicles and the sweat glands which also act as additional sources of epithelium.

When injuries extend to a partial thickness depth, potential sources of epithelium decrease, making a change in the repair process necessary. Repair becomes a combination of (a) granulation, the formation of new connective tissue at the base of a wound, and (b) epithelialization. The granulation proliferates to fill the wound. Epithelium from the borders of the wound and from the few deep remaining structures then bridges the granulation tissue to provide a cover. Healing is still spontaneous, but can take in excess of 3 weeks with large areas.

Once the border between the dermis and the subcutaneous tissue interface is breached, an injury is considered to be of a full thickness depth. The healing processes are too slow to support closure of the wound within a relatively short time, so that repair by skin graft is required.

Grafting is performed on those sites deemed to be of such a depth that spontaneous healing will not occur within 14–21 days, if at all. Only donated skin can provide a permanent repair for the wound. A graft has to be placed on a clean recipient site with an adequate blood supply to promote healing. The area may have to be prepared by escharotomy, excision or debridement of non-viable tissue before a graft is applied. Split thickness grafts which range from 0.006–0.021 in (0.152–0.533 mm) are applied. Where an extensive area is to be covered and/or there is limited donor tissue, split thickness grafts can be meshed.

The outcome of healing is thus dependent on the depth of the original injury. Problems arise for patients when the depth of injury is uncertain. In these deeper wounds the outcome of spontaneous healing may be of poor quality with considerable scarring.

A clinical description of hypertrophic scars

Clinically, hypertrophic scars present as being 'red, raised and rigid'. Those caused by burns have several unique characteristics, including their location and onset. They are commonly found at the border of skin grafts and in wounds of mixed or partial thickness depths. They do not form until the site has epithelialized. Initially the area is flat and smooth and can remain so for up to 4 months. Vascular activity in the area is higher than in surrounding tissue for many months. The area can remain red or *hyperaemic* for an indefinite period. This hyperaemia gradually diminishes, starting at the scar edges. The mature scar eventually pales to a lighter tone than that of surrounding skin. The superficial dermis may be thin and fragile with a decreased elasticity and a reduced tolerance to stretch, and can remain hypersensitive.

Keloid compared with hypertrophic scars

Hypertrophic scars are often mistakenly referred to as keloid(s). However, they have several characteristics which differentiate them. Keloid scars are described as thick scar tissue of the human skin that are produced by excessive amounts of collagen deposited over prolonged periods. They develop gradually following even small skin wounds, and are accompanied by itchiness or *pruritus*. They are not generally painful, and it is usually their cosmetic appearance which causes patients to seek medical advice. The most commonly affected body areas are the pre-sternal region, the back and posterior neck, followed by the ears, shoulders, front of the chest and beard areas. In the chest they can assume a characteristic butterfly shape. They also have a collagen content higher than that found in hypertrophic scars. However, their primary distinguishing feature is that they extend beyond the confines of the original wound. Keloid scars also differ significantly from hypertrophic scars in that the latter will spontaneously soften and flatten with time, whereas keloid scars can remain elevated indefinitely.

A comparison of normal and hypertrophic dermis

The differences between normal and hypertrophic dermis are readily apparent. The contrast begins immediately with the lack of smoothness and the disrupted appearance of hypertrophic skin. While collagen occurs in bundles in normal dermis, it lacks this uniformity in hypertrophic scars. Instead the collagen appears in sworls which adhere together and form nodules. These nodules are seen scattered throughout the wound area, including the deep dermis. Interstitial space is virtually absent, causing disruptions to the course of individual collagen filaments. There is also evidence of fibre-to-fibre fusion which is not seen in normal dermis.

The incidence of hypertrophic scarring

A review of current research suggests that several clinical factors can act as predictors of the occurrence of hypertrophic scarring.

Predictors of hypertrophic scar formation

- **Race.** Blacks are seen to develop wound problems twice as frequently as Whites.

- **Healing time.** There is a greater occurrence of problems the longer it takes a wound to heal, especially where this is greater than 21 days

- **Body location.** The chest, upper arms and feet appear especially prone to hypertrophy when healing is spontaneous

- **Grafting.** When wound sites are grafted, scarring occurs more frequently in young patients than in adults. The head, neck and buttock regions appear more prone to developing hypertrophic scars following grafting than other body parts

The variables present in burned patients that could be used to predict hypertrophy, post-healing, have been analysed by several researchers. One study included 100 patients with 245 separate wound sites. The authors of this study recognized that many wounds go through a phase of hyperaemia and elevation before they revert into normal, flat, mature scars. Hence, they defined hypertrophy as an elevation greater than 2 cm in diameter. They found that 26% of the 245 wound sites were elevated, and that this involved 38% of the patients in the study. The variables they considered included: patient age, race, location of burn and the length of time necessary for the wound to heal spontaneously.

Their results indicated that the incidence of wound problems was twice as high in Blacks as in Whites, especially when healing time was greater than 10 days. They were surprised to find no correlation between age and wound problems, having considered that younger patients would have a higher skin tension with a subsequent tendency towards proliferation in the healing process. They found healing time to be the most important indicator of future wound problems. For example, where wound healing time was greater than 21 days, there was a 78% incidence of hypertrophy. For those wounds that healed spontaneously, the chest, upper extremities and feet were found to be especially prone to hypertrophy. The hand, face and neck regions were more likely to heal without problems.

Grafted wounds have also been found to develop hypertrophic scars. One study which followed up 70 patients that had been grafted found that 36% developed serious scarring in one or more sites. Blacks had a higher incidence than Whites, but both these groups were less affected than paediatric patients. For those patients that had undergone excision of the wound site up to 14 days post-injury, there was a lower incidence of problems than in those grafted after. The findings of this study indicated that a greater number of problems occurred in the head, neck and buttock regions, whereas the extremities and trunk did best. Donor sites were not without their problems, although they were significantly less affected than recipient areas.

The management of hypertrophic scarring

At present there is no known reliable method for predicting the occurrence of hypertrophic scarring and no known method for its prevention. Therefore, the main aim in the management of the hypertrophic scarred area is to minimize the effects of the hypertrophy on the appearance and function of the affected area.

The management of hypertrophic scarring has been a priority of treatment regimens for burn injuries from the earliest days of burn care. Early methods of counteracting the contractile forces in healing burn wounds included traction to the wound site and immobilization of the affected area. These methods are still included in the more acute phases of burn care today, but are not considered efficient long-term management methods for several reasons.

First, burn wound healing and scar formation is a lengthy process, often lasting months. Immobilization and traction have been found to have little permanent influence on the contraction of a healing area once they are discontinued. Secondly, a patient's ability to engage in functional activities is decreased throughout a course of this type of treatment. Patients may also experience considerable discomfort.

Pressure therapy

The application of mechanical pressure is the standard treatment used to minimize the effects of hypertrophic scarring. The use of pressure derives from an early surgical principle, in which the use of bandages and splints was observed to be beneficial, more than 50 years ago.

Methods of pressure application

Several methods of pressure application have been documented. They include the use of open-cell adhesive sponge, splints, bandaging, and elasticated garments. Elasticated or *pressure garments* have become the most commonly used method to manage hypertrophic scars for reasons outlined in the next box.

Pressure garments are used to manage hypertrophic scars because

- they are an easy device to apply
- they are minimally disruptive to activity
- they are available commercially or through skilled technicians
- they can be used to prevent and correct deformity
- they can decrease the need for corrective surgery

However, pressure exerted by garments has been found to vary and appears to be dependent on three factors highlighted below.

Factors which influence the pressure exerted by garments

- Shape of the body parts
- Type and age of the fabric used
- Design and fit of the garment

Shape of the body part

The shape of the underlying body contours is an important influence because the greater the degree of curvature, the greater the pressure exerted. This means that it is easier to apply pressure to certain body parts such as the limbs, rather than to less rounded areas such as the chest wall, pectoral and facial areas.

Type and age of the fabric used

The amount of pressure (measured in mmHg with a pressure manometer) has been found to vary in body locations when garments were made by different technicians, and between different types of fabric, e.g. Lycra or Tubigrip.

Design and fit of the garment

Clinical observation would suggest that garments which fit the patient well and provide a consistent application of pressure appear to produce satisfactory clinical results more often than those that do not.

Pressure garments can be applied as soon as a wound has healed. They are typically used 24 hours a day with no more than two half-hour breaks daily for hygiene purposes. This treatment regimen may be delayed where open areas on the wound site remain or when the epidermis is particularly thin and/or fragile. This is necessary as the shearing force of donning a garment can contribute to further skin breakdown, delaying the wound healing process.

A problem arises when applying pressure where there are prominent elevated ridges on the scar surface. Imagine, if you will, looking down at a series of mountain peaks from your seat in an aircraft. You are going to try and cover those peaks with a huge blanket. You are likely to find that while the whole range is covered, the blanket actually only touches the highest peaks. The valleys between these peaks are not in contact with the blanket. The same thing can occur on a highly contoured scar surface. Although it is relatively simple to apply pressure to elevations of scar tissue, the area between them can be neglected. This allows hypertrophy to continue in these areas. Depending on the size of the area affected, devices known as conformers can be made to fill these spaces. Materials used for this include sponge, Plastazote or silastic elastomer. They are generally worn next to the skin and held in place by the garment.

Complications of pressure therapy

Pressure therapy is not without its complications (Leung *et al.*, 1984). Those known include swelling, blistering and an adverse effect on growing children. As human tissue is viscoelastic, it will become deformed after sustained pressure. Biomechanical principles need to be considered when applying pressure to preserve the body's natural contours, i.e. convexities and concavities like the metacarpal arch and the transverse diameter of the thoracic cage. Padding can be used under garments to fill concavities so that the surface diameter is decreased, and a more even distribution of pressure is encouraged.

Biomechanical forms of treatment

Stretching a scar and moving a joint through its full range of movement several times daily are biomechanical forms of treatment used to prevent contraction of scar tissue by encouraging normal alignment of newly formed collagen fibres. These methods are used in acute burn care. Depending on the severity of the thermal insult, the patient is likely to adopt a position of flexion as this offers the greatest comfort. Healing wounds will contract in conformity with this position, causing the patient greater long-term functional difficulties. Stretching and joint ranging are performed several times daily. The gains made from this form of treatment are usually maintained by positioning devices so that the maximum surface area of a healing wound is maintained. Disadvantages of this treatment are that it is time consuming, labour intensive and often painful for the patient. Continuous passive motion machines (CPMs) have been found helpful in dealing with these problems, as patients appear to have an increased pain tolerance when movement is regular and consistent. Once a patient is well enough, they will be encouraged to do this themselves as often as possible.

Surgical management

Surgical management techniques include excision of scar tissue and z-plasty.

Excision

This in itself has not been found to prevent a re-proliferation of scar tissue, particularly in the case of keloid. Therefore, it is now typically followed by grafting of the site and the application of pressure where necessary.

Z-plasty

This is a surgical procedure used to release contracture from matured scar tissue. It is also used to soften and thin scars and scar infiltrated tissue. Incisions are made at 60° angles in the wound's lines of tension so that newly formed blood vessels will align parallel to these lines. This encourages a more normal configuration of new collagen fibres. Z-plasty has been found useful in scars as old as 25 years (Longacre *et al.*, 1976). In these cases there was a reappearance of unit collagen and elastic fibres which in turn contributed to a more normal dermal composition.

Silicone gel sheets and splints

Silicone gel sheets are being used once a wound has healed spontaneously or when a graft is well established. Their mode of action is not known but is thought likely to involve both hydration of the stratum corneum and the release of low-molecular-weight silicone fluid. These sheets have been found to work best when applied early or to the younger scar. They are secured to the skin surface in a number of ways including taping, bandaging or under pressure garments. Their size, 4 in × 4 in (100 mm × 100 mm) makes them impractical to apply to large areas.

A recent innovation is the development of a means of fabricating splints from silicone which are worn by patients much like pressure garments. A major advantage of these silicone splints includes the fact that they can be moulded to apply consistent pressure in highly contoured body parts like the face and neck. They also appear to be cosmetically unobtrusive. Possible disadvantages of this method of pressure application might include that a high level of technical expertise and training is needed both to make plaster moulds of the scarred area as well as the actual splint(s).

Adhesive contact media

Hypafix, a surgical retention dressing, has been combined with Silastic elastomer to form a product called Elastofix. Elastofix can be applied immediately to fix a new graft to its site and thus has the advantage of early application, which allows it to work to prevent the development of hypertrophic scars. It has also been used correctively once hypertrophy has commenced. Contact media are thought to work by mimicking the action of the stratum corneum, 'reducing water vapour transmission and thereby restoring homeostasis to the burned skin' (Davey *et al.*, 1991). A major clinical benefit of this technique is that treatment time can be shortened by several weeks or months. Further research is required to clarify the mode of action of contact media and to compare it with other forms of treatment. One practical disadvantage for patients is likely to centre on changing the Elastofix, and another the restrictions its use may place on functional activities.

Two theories which suggest why pressure therapy is effective

Keywords

Stasis. A decrease or halt in the flow of body fluids

Blanching. The initial loss of colour owing to decreased blood supply

Hypoxia. Low oxygen content in the blood

Gamma globulins. Protein found in plasma

The *hypoxia theory* is used to explain the effects of pressure on healing burn wounds. The immediate response of the dermis to pressure is a superficial vascular blanching. Pressure also serves to accentuate an already present condition of stasis. Hypoxia is therefore increased to a point where fibroblast activity slows. This in turn impinges on the production of collagen. This process is thought to account for the softening of and decrease in mass of hypertrophic scars under pressure and thereby promotes faster maturation (Kischer *et al.*, 1975).

An alternative theory suggests that scar remodelling may be inhibited by the presence of high levels of gamma globulins. Therefore, pressure therapy may be effective as it decreases the blood flow to the trauma site and thus decreases the availability of gamma globulins. Hence, remodelling would occur at a more rapid pace when pressure is applied. Pressure therapy therefore is not considered to exert influence on the ultrastructure of new scar tissue. It does, however, have an influence on the number of cells, particularly myofibroblasts, present in any given area of scar. This in turn may alter the efficacy or distribution of enzymatic products in a manner which favours nodule breakdown (Baur *et al.*, 1976).

Efficacy of pressure therapy

The effectiveness of pressure therapy is largely determined by visual and tactile assessment of whether the dermis of the mature scar is as flat as that of the surrounding skin. The results of one study of 227 scars treated with pressure and assessed in this way are summarized in the box below.

Effectiveness of pressure therapy

- Nearly one-quarter of scars had an *excellent* result, one-half were considered *good*, while one-quarter were *fair*. Less than 1% had *poor* results.

- The head, neck, foot and leg had a higher incidence of *fair* results.

- The arms, hands and trunk produced *better* results

It was once thought that 25 mmHg of pressure was needed to influence the scarring process. However, research evidence suggests that this pressure is seldom achieved and is unnecessary, and in some cases can be detrimental for reasons previously mentioned.

There is also evidence to suggest that the range of effective pressure resides between 5 and 15 mmHg. It also appears that the *consistency* rather than the *amount* of pressure applied to a scar site may be the more important determinant of treatment success.

The construction methods advocated in this manual produce garments which have yielded clinical success over a 20-year history. However, as mentioned previously, the pressure exerted by garments is known to vary with the design and construction method used, the type and age of fabric used, body location and patient posture. A simple way to monitor the pressure being exerted over scar sites is the use of a pressure manometer when the patient visits the clinic for the initial fitting of garments and any follow-up visits. Figure 1.4 shows one type of pressure manometer. These devices are available from commercial manufacturers, one of which is listed in Appendix I. It is recommended that the reader considers means of measuring pressure objectively, particularly where this is a new area of practice to you.

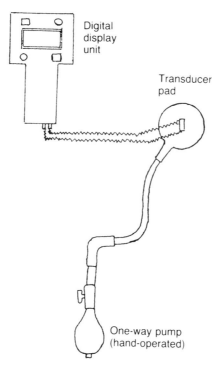

Figure 1.4 **Pressure manometer**

Pressure therapy treatment protocol

Prior to the wound site healing, pressure is applied indirectly through the use of splints and bandages. Following healing, pressure is applied through the use of tubular elasticated bandage or pressure garments, particularly to those patients who fall into the risk categories described earlier.

For those patients with one or more of the risk factors present, pressure is best applied prophylactically, i.e. as soon as new skin cover has formed and become established. This essentially means that most patients are discharged from the burns unit with some type of pressure garment. However, because new dermis is fragile and susceptible to breaks and tears, those clinicians providing the pressure therapy service have to judge the patient's skin tolerance to the shearing forces of pressure garments. If Lycra garments cannot be tolerated, pressure can be applied initially with tubular elasticated stockinette for limbs, and bandaging or splints for torso, axillae and hand locations.

Patients may undergo dramatic changes initially on discharge from hospital. Increasing weight or muscle bulk and changes in oedema are common factors which influence the pressure exerted by garments on the body and which will need to be monitored fairly closely. Our patients typically have an outpatient appointment with the plastic surgeon 2 weeks after discharge, at which time they are also assessed for any changes required in their pressure therapy. Patients and their families are also advised on signs and symptoms which could indicate potential problems. A sample advice sheet is given in Appendix II.

Once the patient's weight, muscle bulk and oedema have stabilized and the new dermis is well established, each patient is provided with three sets of the particular Lycra garments they require. This is necessary as the garments have to be worn for 23 hours per day and laundered by hand daily. The patient is advised on the care of garments to protect the elastic fibres, and thus the consistency with which pressure is applied to a scar. The garments are usually replaced every 6–12 weeks, depending on the patient's activity level, etc. Once the clinician is satisfied that the scars are being well managed, i.e. receiving consistent pressure, are supple, and the patient's contours are stable, the patient needs only to attend for follow-up appointments on a 3-monthly basis. Patients are encouraged to call the clinic when they require replacement garments in the interim, which are then mailed out to them.

Patients wear pressure garments for the entire period the scars remain active, i.e. in most cases 12 months. Once the hyperaemia has subsided, and the scar site has flattened, pressure can be discontinued. With some patients this may mean removing the garments for short periods initially and observing the scar site for any increase in elevation, colour or pruritus in the area.

Application of pressure to facial locations is a topical clinical issue. Luckily, burns to the face occur far less frequently than in other body locations. Pressure garments are becoming less the treatment of choice for facial scars for a number of reasons, particularly with children. First, the face is highly contoured, with peak pressures occurring on anatomical prominences like the chin. Where this pressure continues long term, anatomical deformity has been observed. Secondly, given that there is little skeletal support underlying the cheeks, pressure is very difficult to apply consistently. Thirdly, many patients find that the benefits of facial helmets are not balanced with the discomfort they can cause. The treatment protocol is altered for facial scars, such that the patient is advised to use the garment for short periods or at night only. Alternative management methods, discussed earlier, are used where appropriate.

In addition to the use of garments, patients are advised to massage their scar sites twice daily with a non-allergenic cream, in order to keep the area supple. Ranging and stretching exercises are also prescribed where necessary, in conjunction with the use of pressure therapy, to keep scar sites from contracting. The following box highlights the main points of a pressure therapy treatment regimen.

Pressure therapy treatment regimen

- Pressure is applied as soon as a wound site has healed

- If the new skin is too fragile to withstand the shearing forces of Lycra pressure garments, then alternatives like tubular elastic stockinette should be used

- Patients are instructed that pressure must be applied for 23 hours a day, with two hygiene breaks

- Patients should be discharged from acute care using some form of pressure therapy where possible. If pressure garments are used, two sets are usually supplied

- Follow-up should take place on a weekly basis for the first month to monitor changes in oedema, muscle bulk and skin tolerance. Alterations to the pressure devices being used should be made accordingly

- Follow-up can then be done on a twice- or once-monthly basis depending on the status of the wound sites

- Garments should be replaced as needed; this is usually every 8–10 weeks. Patients are usually supplied with four sets of garments once stabilized, to ensure consistent pressure application

- As a scar sight flattens and/or fades towards a lighter skin colour, pressure therapy can gradually decrease in time, for example only at night and, finally, not at all. The patient should be shown how to monitor the status of their own scar site for redness and itchiness. If this recurs, the garments should be reapplied

2

Stages in garment construction

Designing and making pressure garments is a technical skill to which the old maxim 'practice makes perfect' applies. You will need to have knowledge of basic mathematics and some sewing experience. Before making garments for patients it is advisable to make several for yourself and colleagues. Try wearing them for increasing lengths of time to get an appreciation of the practical problems patients may have

The great majority of patients are compliant with their pressure therapy for the entire treatment period. Many report immediate relief from pruritus when pressure is applied. The results of pressure application are usually readily apparent, particularly when scars are hyperaemic and elevated. This encourages patients' motivation to continue with the treatment. Occasionally, a patient may find the treatment regimen difficult to maintain. At these times, informal counselling or a chat with a fellow patient may be useful. The authors have found that compliance with treatment is more of a problem in hot countries or when the temperature rises locally.

The methods for garment construction recommended in this manual evolved from experience gained by the staff in the Occupational Therapy Department, Withington Hospital, Manchester. A Lycra fabric (No. 25034, from Penn-Nyla Ltd, listed in Appendix I), is typically used to manufacture garments. Given the weight and extensibility of this fabric, a mathematical formula was devised to be used in pattern drafting. Basically, all circumferential measurements are multiplied by 0.4, and used to draft pattern pieces which are usually half the required width. These pattern pieces are then cut from folded fabric, thus doubling their width. The resulting fabric shape represents 80% of the circumference of its corresponding body part. The fabric in the garment is thus stretched by 20% to exert pressure onto a scar site. Length measurements typically have between one-fifth to one-quarter of their total deducted.

This construction method has yielded consistent results over the years. The use of this mathematical formula ensures that a uniform amount of fabric is deducted throughout a garment. The pressure exerted is thus consistent, irrespective of which staff member made the garment, as the same pattern pieces and tailoring techniques are used.

Pressure can also be applied with greater consistency when garments are purpose made to individual patient contours. It is an advantage when the person who made a garment fits it to the patient, as minor changes are often needed to pattern pieces, given the changes that can occur in the human body on a weekly (or even a daily!) basis. By fitting a garment on a patient, the clinician can see immediately where garments need to be altered.

The following box lists the stages involved in garment design and fabrication. Each stage will be described in full.

Pressure garments: stages in design and fabrication

- **Patient measurement**
- **Selection of garment design**
- **Draft pattern**
- **Fabric selection**
- **Cut pattern from fabric**
- **Sew garment together**
- **Fit garment to patient**

Patient measurement

Use a tape measure that will follow body contours closely. Tape measures which are very stiff or which have long metal tips at either end may lead to inaccurate measurements, particularly in small body parts. All measurements are taken in centimetres (cm) to the first decimal place, e.g. 19.1 cm.

In general, two types of measurements are needed to design a pressure garment:

- **those which go around a body part (circumferential measurements)**
- **those which measure the length of a body part (longitudinal measurements)**

Circumferential measurements are multiplied by 0.4, but longitudinal measurements are not quite so straightforward. Generally, one-fifth to one-quarter of the length is deducted from its total, e.g. a forearm length of 20 cm will have between 4 and 5 cm deducted in preparation for pattern drafting. However, this will vary according to

(a) limb size: we have found that wider, longer limbs need less deducted
(b) how firm the underlying body part is, i.e. highly contoured body parts

and/or those with loose or pendulous skin cover usually need less deducted from their length measurements.

In some instances, measurements have to be altered 'by eye' or judgement alone. For example, when fitting a sleeve into a vest, a measurement is taken from mid-axilla to the base of the lateral aspect of the neck. The angle at which this is drawn on the pattern will rely on your observations of the shoulder's girth, the patient's postural patterns and the site of the scarring. A measurement is taken diagonally from the highest point on the instep, around the heel and back. This will have to be accommodated in pattern drafting and often serves as the starting point for sock patterns, around which the other measurements will have to be plotted.

All measurements are recorded on the *measurement charts* located in each appropriate chapter and in Appendix III.

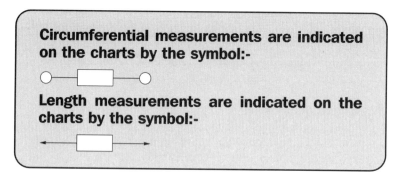

Circumferential measurements are indicated on the charts by the symbol:-

Length measurements are indicated on the charts by the symbol:-

Glove measurements

The hand's size and highly contoured anatomy have necessitated a novel measurement technique. A patient is asked to place the hand, palm down, onto a piece of blank paper with the fingers in slight abduction. Where a patient has difficulty achieving full finger extension, measurements can be taken following stretching exercises. Alternatively, you may have to apply your own hand to the dorsum of the patient's hand to achieve the maximum extension possible. This will also serve to ensure that the hand does not move during measurement. Holding a pencil or narrow point felt tip pen perpendicular to the hand and following the hand's shape closely, trace around the entire outline directly onto the paper. If the pencil is not held exactly perpendicular to the paper, inaccurate measurement will result in a garment that is too tight. Accuracy is especially important at the web spaces between fingers.

Design considerations

Once you have taken your patient's measurements you will have to decide which type of garment will best serve the purpose. The garment will have to cover the scar well to provide consistent pressure as well as allow the patient to perform daily activities with the minimal hindrance possible. As pressure garments are worn under clothing, they are usually concealed by the patient's own clothes.

Several factors have to be borne in mind when selecting which type of garment you will make:

1. In order to exert adequate pressure over a scar site, garments should extend 5 cm above and below the scar site(s). This is also necessary as garments are gradually flared at each end or opening to ensure that normal blood and fluid movement within the body is not disrupted. Hence, a mid-calf scar could be managed with a below-knee sock, while a scar at the knee joint crease would need a garment which extended to the mid-thigh at least.

2. Garments should not cause or contribute to oedema. Where oedema is or could become a problem, garments should be extended to the distal end of limbs. For example, a mid-forearm scar could normally be managed with a below-elbow sleeve, but if the arm or hand is oedematous a long glove would be made. Similarly, a newly healing leg wound site will probably need to be managed with the foot incorporated into the garment design to minimize the effect of dependent oedema.

3. Pressure garments, because they are close fitting, are susceptible to 'rolling' when the patient moves. This is especially so for garments which cross joints and for lower limb garments. To overcome this problem, one simple solution is to sew wide (i.e. 2.5 cm) elastic inside the proximal (or top) end of all garments which are used on limbs alone, and/or the distal (or bottom) end of jackets and vests at the waistband to keep them from rolling up. With active small children it is helpful to add an extension to the back of a jacket or vest which passes between the legs (over diapers or underwear) and fastens to the front of the garment with Velcro. This serves as an 'anchor' for the garments and stops them rolling up.

4. The amount of pressure exerted by garments is related to the degree of curvature of the underlying body parts. A lower degree

of curvature means that pressure can be exerted more consistently. In order to decrease the curvature of body parts, padding is often used under garments. For instance, if we consider a cross-section of the mid-torso, the abdomen is curved while the back has a hollow. Thus the pressure exerted by garments to scars located in this hollow would be minimal if at all. Using a piece of padding or foam in this area ensures that pressure is exerted evenly. Padding is often required for axillae and upper chest scars.

5. When scars are very lumpy or have thick ridges on them, the pressure exerted by a garment will not reach the dips or troughs between these ridges. Pads are often not pliant enough to fill small dips. Conformers can be made from silastic elastomer which are then made to cover these scars and are worn under the garments. Silastic elastomer is a product made by Dow Corning Ltd and consists of two components which are liquid. When mixed together and poured over a scar they harden to form a rubbery mould of the scar's surface underneath while remaining smooth on top. They are fairly durable and can be washed for hygiene purposes without damage.

Gloves are usually made with the fingertips left open so as not to impair sensation. For patients with scars which extend to the fingertips, these openings can be closed. With extensive scars, other management techniques are also likely to be used, e.g. exercises and massage.

The patient's ability to put on and take off the garments will need to be considered at this stage. For patients with extensive scars, particularly in the hands, or where there is decreased strength and range of movement, adapted garments may be necessary. This could include the use of extra zippers, Velcro fastenings or the use of lighter fabric. If the patient has assistance from a carer or family member, they will need to be shown the best ways to assist the patient.

The charts at the end of this chapter are included to help you in garment design selection. Garment indications, types and the number of both pattern and fabric pieces required to assemble each garment are listed.

Drafting patterns

All patterns are drafted onto blank sheets of paper. We have found a large roll of general-purpose paper (e.g. newsprint or brown parcel paper) useful for large pattern pieces, e.g. leggings, jackets and full-length sleeves.

Length lines are always drawn with a ruler. Circumferential measurements are plotted from these lines.

Remember

- All circumferential measurements are multiplied by 0.4
- All lengths have between one-fifth and one-quarter of their total deducted

Pattern pieces, with a few exceptions, represent half the amount of fabric needed, so are usually placed on doubled or folded fabric. This is done to minimize the number of seams needed in a garment and so promote consistent pressure exertion.

Fold symbols

The diagrams in this manual will have a fold symbol to indicate that a pattern piece should be placed on a folded piece of fabric before cutting it out. The symbol looks like this:

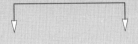

Once the patient's contours, e.g. weight, muscle bulk and oedema, are fairly stable, pattern pieces can be reused to supply new garments. It is useful to record the patient's name and the date the measurements were taken on each piece, as well as whether it is a **R**ight or **L**eft garment (**R** and **L** being convenient abbreviations).

Fabric selection

We usually keep a selection of two or three types of fabric which vary in their weight and extensibility. The fabric used for garments is chosen according to how elevated the patient's scars are, the fragility of the skin covering the scars, how well the patient is able to don garments and the patient's tolerance. Lycra suppliers are listed in Appendix I. They are usually willing to provide samples which may be helpful in deciding which fabrics you will stock.

Elastic fibres deteriorate with time, even when stored on a shelf. If you are treating small numbers of patients, or only infrequently, it is as well to order fabric is amounts of just a few metres at a time.

If pressure therapy is started before scars become too elevated or established, it is possible to manage them with the lighter fabrics which patients find more comfortable. It is usual to start pressure therapy with the lighter fabrics and so increase the patient's tolerance to pressure. However, garments made from the lighter fabrics will deteriorate faster and therefore need replacing more frequently. The clinician will need to consider the patient's needs and the resources available.

Fabric

The fabric typically used to make pressure is Lycra. This is woven such that there can be variation in the elastic : nylon ratio, which consequently alters the fabric weight, stretch and extensibility. The fabric we have found to provide consistent results for a wide range of applications has a 72% nylon: 28% Lycra ratio. This is available from Penn-Nyla Ltd (listed in Appendix I), code number 25034. This is a weft-knitted fabric which means that there is a greater stretch in one direction. It is important that this direction of stretch corresponds with the body's circumferential measurements to achieve good pressure application.

Cutting patterns from fabric

Pattern pieces are placed on folded or doubled (two layers) fabric with the elastic fibres of the fabric corresponding with the direction of the circumferential measurements.

Pattern pieces are pinned to the fabric to secure them in place. Avoid using too many pins as they tend to break the elastic fibres of the Lycra fabric.

No seam allowances are made with pressure garments, so pattern outlines should be followed exactly when cutting them out.

Sewing the garment

Once all the pattern pieces are cut out, garments are assembled. All seams in pressure garments are located on the *outside of garments*. As garments are so close fitting, having the seams on the inside would increase the pressure over seam sites.

A very close, narrow zigzag stitch of no more than 0.3 cm is used to join seams. No space between stitches should be visible. Flat seams are used on weight-bearing surfaces, e.g. the volar surface of socks, and when inserting gussets. These are made by overlapping the fabric sections by 0.5 cm and sewing them together. Elastic is inserted with a well-spaced zigzag stitch. This is referred to in the instructions as a 'long' zigzag stitch.

Some patients find pressure garments uncomfortable at joint creases, particularly the elbows and axillae, which can also be a site of skin breakdown. A piece of absorbent, stretchy cotton fabric, e.g. T-shirt material, can be sewn inside garments over joint areas before sewing the side seams together. Cotton material will also absorb perspiration which increases garment comfort.

Inserting a zipper into a pressure garment

1. Place the closed zipper onto the *right* side of the fabric (Figure 2.1). The precise location of the zip will depend on the garment design. Refer to individual pattern instructions as necessary.
2. Sew along the sides and the closed end of the zipper using a 0.3 cm zigzag stitch.

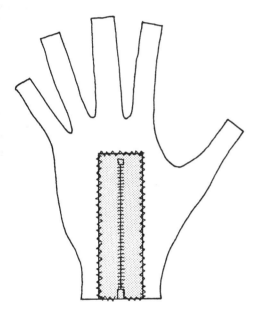

Figure 2.1 **Zipper sewn onto right side of fabric**

3. Cut away the fabric underneath the zipper, close to the inside edge of the seams.
4. Insert a backing strip behind the zipper (Figure 2.2). This is made from a piece of Lycra fabric, cut to measure the length of the zipper and twice its width. Fold the fabric in half lengthways and position it to cover the back of the zipper.
5. Match the open edges of the backing strip to one zipper seam and sew into place, leaving the folded edge free.

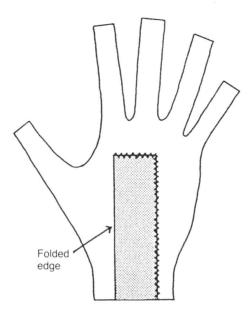

Folded
edge

Figure 2.2 **Backing strip on inside of palm piece**

Inserting gussets

Gussets are V-shaped, 1 cm strips of Lycra fabric. They are inserted into the finger and thumb web spaces on the dorsum of gloves and mittens. They are necessary to:

(a) accommodate finger girth, and
(b) apply pressure to web spaces.

Gussets are made from a right-angled template (Figure 2.3) – see also Appendix IV for a copy of the template pattern. Templates should be cut from a rigid material, such as metal or stiff plastic, so that they can be held firmly in place when placed on fabric.

1. Place the template onto the Lycra so that the direction of fabric stretch corresponds to the width of the template. Draw around the template directly onto the fabric (Figure 2.4). Cut out carefully.
2. A 1 cm slit is made in the centre of each web space on the dorsal piece of fabric of the glove/mitten.
3. The gusset is pinned on top of the dorsal piece of fabric so that the outside point of the V matches the base of the slit. These two pieces will overlap and should be sewn with a flat seam of 0.3 cm width (Figure 2.5). When sewing the gussets into position, it may be easiest to sew two separate seams from the point of the V to each fingertip. As your sewing skill improves, you may find that you can insert gussets with a single seam, starting from a fingertip.

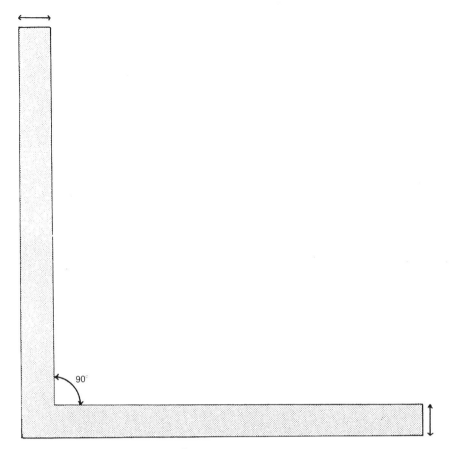

Figure 2.3 **Glove gusset template**

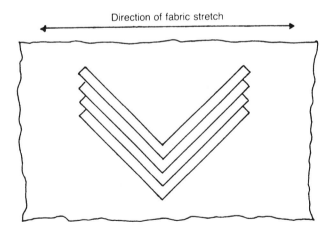

Direction of fabric stretch

Figure 2.4 **Drawing around the gusset template on fabric**

4. With wrong sides together, match the web space of the palmar
    piece with the inside edge of the gusset. Sew together with a 0.3
    cm zigzag seam.

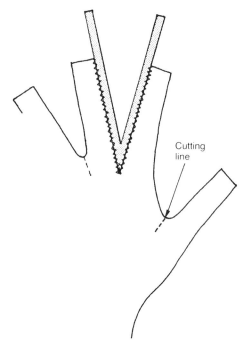

Cutting
line

Figure 2.5 **Gusset sewn to fabric with a flat seam**

Elastic

Use 2.5 cm wide elastic which has one soft side, where possible. This side should face the patient's skin. Elastic is sewn around the inside edge of openings when indicated. It is always sewn into place using a long zigzag stitch of 0.5 cm width.

Fitting the garment

Patients should be reassured that garments will feel snug. Assistance will be needed to don garments when they are new, but they do get easier to put on with time. To ensure that they are not too tight, the clinician should check by pulling along various garment seams. With the exception of gloves, you should be able to pull seams between 1 and 2 cm away from the skin. You should also be able to insert a full fingertip under each opening in garments.

Adjustments can be made to the garment when it is fitted. It may be necessary to alter seams or lengths at this time. Any changes made to the garment should be noted on the pattern piece.

The patient should remain in the clinic for at least half an hour on the first fitting session. Observe the colour of the extremities for anoxia (the skin will take on a bluish tinge), and have the patient report any paraesthesia (sensation of 'pins and needles'). The patient should be advised never to alter or cut the garment personally, as this will release pressure in one spot but which will act like a tourniquet in other parts, impairing blood and fluid movement. Releasing pressure in this way may also cause oedema of the extremities. For this reason, patients should also be taught to look for holes in garments. If they cannot be mended, the garment may have to be discarded.

It is important that you read through the full set of instructions before making any garment, to familiarize yourself with the stages of construction.

Checklist

Once you have made and fitted a garment, check the following points:

- Ask the patient how it feels and note any area of discomfort, which you should try to address

- Look for breaks in the seams. These must be mended immediately, as they can act as a tourniquet by increasing the pressure in a band around the limb

- Check the patient's extremities for changes in oedema, skin colour, temperature and/or sensation

- Ensure that you can get your full fingertip under any opening in the garment

- Ensure all seams can easily be pulled between 1 and 2 cm away from the skin, except in the case of gloves where it is unnecessary

- Check the joint creases so that movements will not cause friction and subsequent skin breakdown

- Make sure the garment covers the scar site by at least 5 cm in all directions

- Instruct the patient on the care of scars and garments

- Supply two or three sets of garments initially and renew as required (usually every 8–10 weeks)

The following chapters provide detailed instructions for designing and making pressure garments for specific body locations. A number of abbreviations are used on diagrams and in the text to indicate specific anatomical parts. The box below highlights these.

Body locations

Hand

P	Palm
D	Dorsum (back of the hand)
CMC	Carpometacarpal joint (at the base of the thumb)
MCP	Metacarpophalangeal joint (knuckle)
PIP	Proximal interphalangeal joint (the first joint in each finger above the knuckle)
DIP	Distal interphalangeal joint (the second joint in each finger above the knuckle)

Arm

W	Wrist
E	Elbow
AE	Above elbow
BE	Below elbow
A	Axilla (armpit)

Skull

TMJ	Temporomandibular joint (forms the hinge between the upper and lower jaw)

Trunk

W	Waist
B	Buttock

Leg

K	Knee
AK	Above knee
B/K	Below knee
A	Ankle
H	Heel
T	Toe

Garment indications

For scar sites in the following body locations:

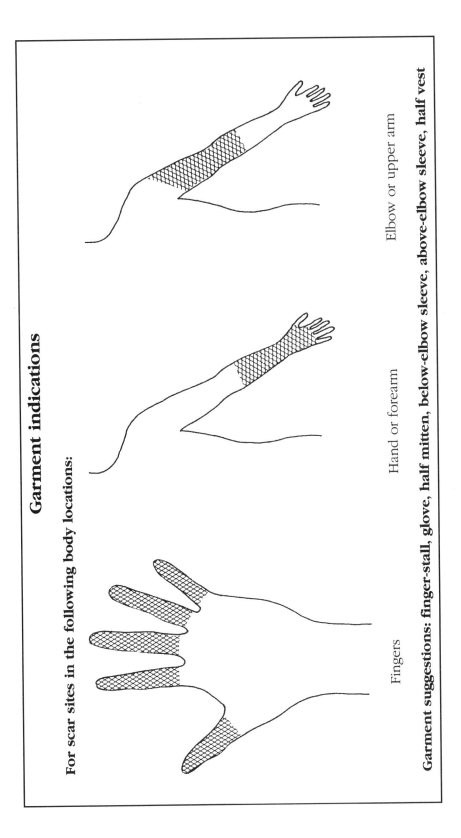

Fingers   Hand or forearm   Elbow or upper arm

Garment suggestions: finger-stall, glove, half mitten, below-elbow sleeve, above-elbow sleeve, half vest

Garment indications

For scar sites in the following body locations:

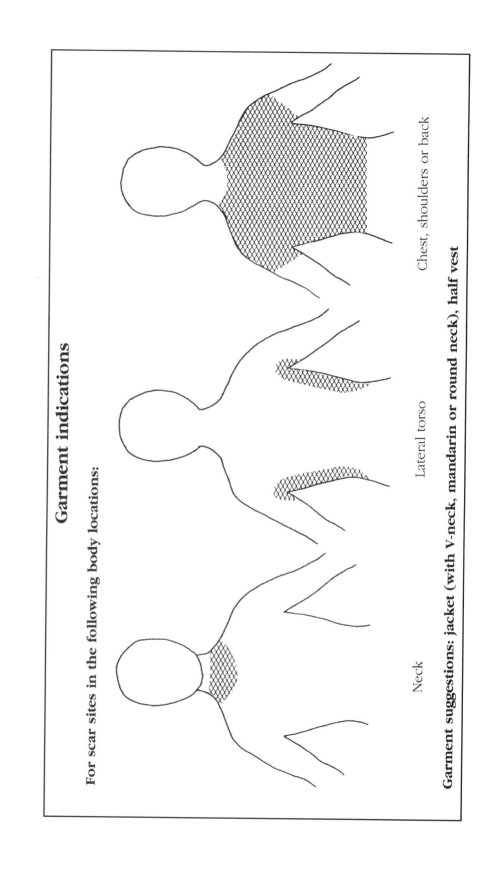

Neck   Lateral torso   Chest, shoulders or back

Garment suggestions: jacket (with V-neck, mandarin or round neck), half vest

Garment indications

For scar sites in the following body locations:

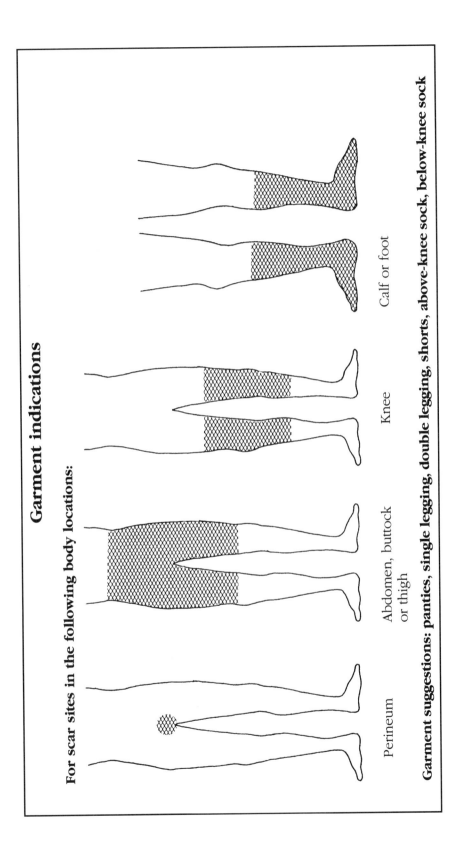

Perineum   Abdomen, buttock   Knee   Calf or foot
                  or thigh

Garment suggestions: panties, single legging, double legging, shorts, above-knee sock, below-knee sock

Garment indications

For scar sites in the following body locations:

Face or scalp   Chin or neck

Garment suggestions: chin strap, mask

3

Upper limb garments

It is important that you read Chapter 2 before you begin making any pressure garment. Construction methods for the following garments are described in this chapter:

> **Finger-stall**
>
> **Half mitten**
>
> **Glove**
>
> **Below-elbow sleeve**
>
> **Above-elbow sleeve**

FINGER-STALL

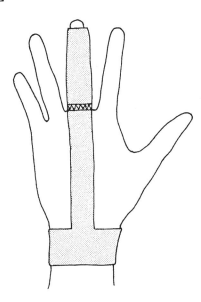

1. Measurements

1a. The patient places the hand, palm down, onto a piece of blank paper.

1b. Trace around the finger, holding the pencil perpendicular to the paper.

2. Drafting the pattern

2a. As gussets are not used in this pattern, allowance has to be made for the finger circumference. Add a uniform 0.5 cm to each side of the finger outline to form the pattern. These lines should then be tapered at the fingertip.

2b. Draw a straight line across the pattern at the fingertip end. Remember that the ends of pressure garments on the fingers are left open so as not to impair sensitivity.

2c. Join the two length lines of the pattern with another straight line at the base of the finger. This completes the pattern (Figure 3.1). Cut it out carefully.

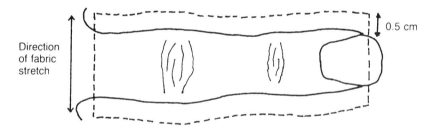

Figure 3.1 **Finger-stall pattern lines**

3. Cutting the fabric

3a. Pin the pattern onto a doubled piece of fabric. Ensure that the direction of the fabric stretch corresponds with the finger width, rather than its length.

3b. Cut the fabric out, following the pattern lines accurately.

3c. Remove the pattern.

4. Sewing the garment

4a. Sew up the side seams of the finger-stall, leaving both ends open.

5. Modifications

5a. Should the garment need to be secured, straps made of Lycra or webbing can be sewn to the base of the garment on the dorsal surface. These should be long enough to secure at the wrist with Velcro or tied (Figure 3.2).

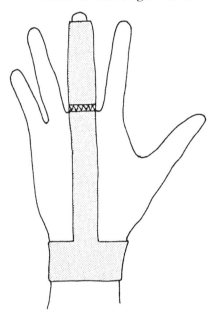

Figure 3.2 **Completed finger-stall**

HALF MITTEN

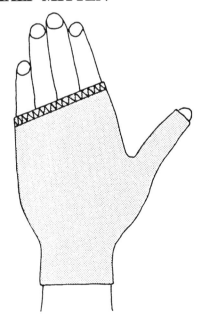

1. Measurements

1a. The patient places the hand, palm down, onto a piece of blank paper. The fingers should be together, with the thumb in slight extension. Ensure that the forearm, wrist and hand are aligned.

1b. Draw around the hand and forearm to approximately 5 cm proximal to the wrist, holding the pencil perpendicular to the paper. It is not necessary to draw round each individual finger.

1c. Mark the position of the PIP joints of the index and little fingers onto the paper. Mark also the CMC joint and the base of the hypothenar eminence.

2. Drafting the pattern

2a. Using a ruler, draw a straight line just below the two marks which indicate the PIP joints. This line will form the top edge of the pattern.

2b. Flare the pattern towards its opening at the wrist. The flare lines should start at approximately the CMC joint of the thumb on one side and the base of the hypothenar eminence on the other side. The size of the flare will depend on the girth of the patient's wrist and forearm (see Chapter 2).

2c. Draw a line across the forearm, to join the flared lines, and to form the bottom edge of the pattern.

2d. Draw a straight line across the tip of the thumb to square it. This completes the pattern (Figure 3.3). Cut it out carefully.

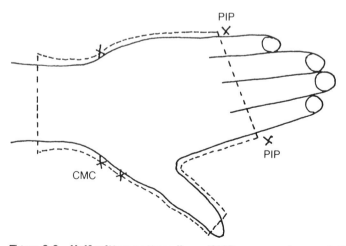

Figure 3.3 **Half mitten pattern lines (CMC, carpometacarpal; PIP, proximal interphalangeal)**

3. Cutting the fabric

3a. Pin the pattern onto a doubled piece of fabric. Ensure that the direction of the fabric stretch corresponds with the hand's width, rather than its length.

3b. Cut the fabric out, following the pattern lines accurately.

3c. Remove the pattern. Use small marks to indicate one of the fabric pieces '**D**' for dorsum and the other '**P**' for palm. You may also need to mark them **L**eft and **R**ight if you are making half mittens for both of the patient's hands.

4. Sewing the garment

4a. Take the fabric piece marked D, and cut a 1 cm slit in the centre of the web space of the thumb. Sew a finger gusset into the web space using a flat seam. Ensure that the point of the 'V' in the gusset matches the end of the slit you have made (see Chapter 2). Trim the end of the gusset to match the top edge of the fabric.

4b. Taking the fabric piece marked P, match the web space with the inside edge of the gusset on the dorsum piece. Pin in place with one pin at the base of the web space. Sew together.

4c. Fold the fabric 0.5 cm along the PIP joint line and sew with a long zigzag stitch to make a small hem.

4d. Sew the side seams. This completes the garment (Figure 3.4).

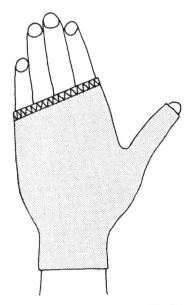

Figure 3.4 **Completed half mitten**

5. Modifications

5a. Occasionally you may need to insert a zipper into a half mitten. This is usually done as the first sewing step. A 12.5 cm zipper is suitable for most adults. The zipper should be closed and sewn onto the outside of the palm piece of fabric. Ensure that the zipper opens from the forearm edge (or bottom) of the garment. Cut away the fabric under the zipper. Sew a 12.5 cm backing strip into place (see Chapter 2).

GLOVE

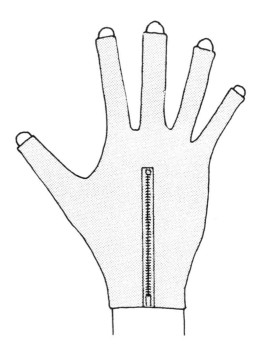

1. Measurements

1a. The patient places the hand, palm down, onto a blank piece of paper. The fingers should be abducted, and the thumb slightly extended. Ensure that the forearm, wrist and hand are aligned.

1b. Draw around the hand and forearm to approximately 5 cm proximal to the wrist, while holding the pen perpendicular to the paper. Ensure that web spaces are accurately drawn.

1c. Mark the location of:

    (i) the CMC and MCP joints of the thumb
    (ii) the MCP joint of the little finger, and
    (iii) the base of the hypothenar eminence of the little finger.

2. Drafting the pattern

2a. Using a ruler, draw a straight line on the pattern across the forearm, 5 cm proximal to the wrist to form the end of the pattern.

2b. Flare the pattern:

   (i) from the marked CMC joint to the forearm line, and
   (ii) from the marked base of the hypothenar eminence to the
        forearm line.

   The size of these flares will usually be approximately 1 cm each,
   but is dependent on the wrist girth of individual patients (see
   Chapter 2).

2c. Next, flare the pattern at the thumb and little finger by 0.5 cm from
   the MCP joints of both to their tips.

2d. Draw straight lines across each finger and thumb tip to square
   them. Mark the pattern **Left** or **Right**. This completes the pattern
   (Figure 3.5). Cut it out carefully.

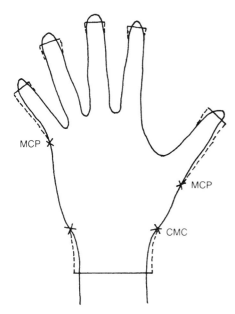

Figure 3.5 **Glove pattern lines**

3. Cutting the fabric

3a. Pin pattern onto a doubled piece of fabric, ensuring that the direction of fabric stretch corresponds with the hand's width and not
   with its length.

3b. Cut the pattern out carefully.

3c. Mark one pattern piece **P**alm and the other **D**orsum.

3d. On the **dorsum** piece only, cut a 1 cm slit in the centre of each web space (Figure 3.6). This makes it easier to sew the gussets into place.

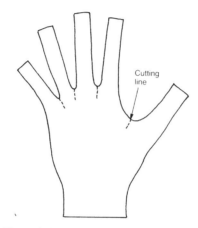

Figure 3.6 **Position of web space slits**

4. Sewing the glove

4a. A 12.5 cm zipper should be centred and sewn to the right side of the palmar piece of fabric. Remember that the zipper should open at the forearm edge of the garment. Cut away the fabric directly under the zipper.

4b. Sew a 12.5 cm backing strip into place (see Chapter 2).

4c. Sew gussets into the web spaces on the D piece of fabric with a flat seam (see Chapter 2).

4d. Sew the D and P pieces together on the little finger side of the glove. Start the seam from the forearm edge and sew down to the fingertip.

4e. For each finger, match the edge of the web space on the P piece with the inside edge of the gusset on the D piece. Pin and sew together.

4f. Trim excess gusset from each fingertip.

4g. Sew final side seam, from the forearm edge to the tip of the thumb.

4h. Once the glove is fitted, mark and trim each finger of the glove so that the patient's fingertips are just visible (Figure 3.7).

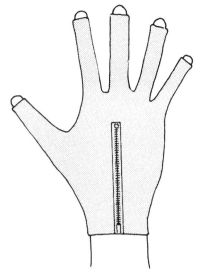

Figure 3.7 **Completed glove**

5. Web spacer

5a. You may encounter patients who have scarring in the web spaces between their fingers. Scarring here can affect hand function quite markedly. A glove may not be adequate to apply pressure to this area on its own. The web spacer shown in Figure 3.8 is made from a wrist cuff of webbing material with a fastening of Velcro (not shown). Lengths of elastic (or Lycra fabric), measured directly on the patient's hand, are sewn to the wrist cuff. The web spacer is worn over the glove as an accessory to it.

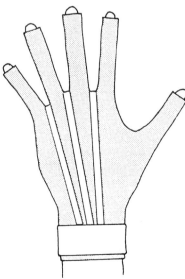

Figure 3.8 **Web spacer shown over glove – dorsal view. Velcro fastener (not shown) is on the palmar aspect of the wrist**

BELOW-ELBOW SLEEVE

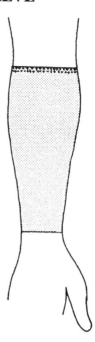

1. Measurement

1a. To make a below-elbow sleeve, use measuring chart number 1 located at the end of this chapter and in Appendix III.

1b. Measure for the length of the sleeve with the elbow extended, from 2 cm below the elbow to the wrist.

1c. Next, take the circumferential measurements in the locations shown on the measuring chart, i.e. approximately 5 cm intervals.

1d. Calculate the pattern measurements by:

    (i) subtracting 15–20% from the length measurement, and
    (ii) multiplying each circumferential measurement by 0.4.

For example, a measured length of 20 cm is shortened by 20%, or 4cm, to 16 cm. A circumferential measurement of 22.8 cm is then multiplied by 0.4 and equals 9.1 cm. These adjusted circumferential measurements are then used to construct your paper pattern.

2. Drafting the pattern

2a. Using a ruler:

    (i) draw a line on the paper to represent the newly calculated length of the sleeve,

(ii) mark one end of this line **W**rist and the other **E**lbow

(iii) use your adjusted circumferential wrist measurement to draw a straight line up from the horizontal line at the wrist end, and

(iv) repeat this for the elbow measurement (Figure 3.9).

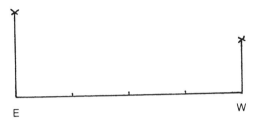

E   W

Figure 3.9 **The length, elbow and wrist lines (E, elbow; W, wrist)**

2b. Mark the other adjusted circumferential measurements onto the pattern, ensuring that they are accurately spaced. It is not necessary to draw lines for these measurements, but simply indicate their locations with a small 'x' (Figure 3.10).

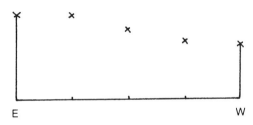

E   W

Figure 3.10 **The plotted circumferential measurements**

2c. Complete the outline of the pattern by connecting these marks with a pencil line. This line should flow smoothly to approximate the contours of the arm.

2d. Flare each end of the pattern slightly, by no more than 1 cm at the wrist and 1.5 cm at the elbow. Mark the length line with a 'fold' symbol. This completes the pattern (Figure 3.11). Cut it out carefully.

3. Cutting the fabric

3a. Pin the pattern onto a folded piece of fabric:

(i) ensuring that the length line is on the fabric fold, and

(ii) ensuring that the direction of stretch of the fabric corresponds with the direction of the circumferential measurements and not with the length.

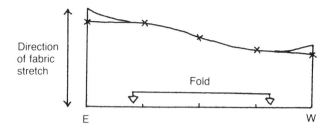

Figure 3.11 **The flared ends of the pattern**

3b. Cut the pattern out, following the lines accurately.

3c. Remove the pattern and unfold the fabric.

4. Sewing the garment

4a. Cut a piece of elastic 1 cm longer than the width of the garment at its top (elbow) end. This will give you a 0.5 cm excess at either edge. Lay the elastic on the fabric so that the top edges of both are flush.

4b. Remember that the elastic is sewn on the inside of the garment, so make sure that the softest side will face the skin (Figure 3.12). Sew this into place.

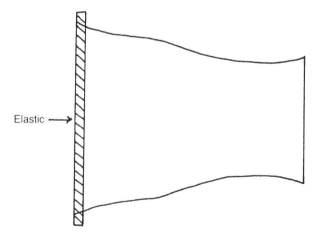

Figure 3.12 **Elastic sewn into elbow end of the sleeve before joining up the main seam**

4c. Fold the fabric lengthways to align the edges and pin together. Starting at the top, sew these edges together. Trim excess elastic to finish. This completes the garment (Figure 3.13).

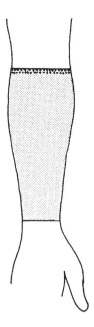

Figure 3.13 **The completed below-elbow sleeve**

5. Modifications

Above-elbow sleeve

The length of the sleeve can be extended as required by taking additional length and circumferential measurements (Figure 3.14).

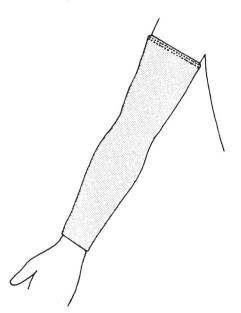

Figure 3.14 **Completed above-elbow sleeve**

Chart No. 1: Below-elbow sleeve

Date ....
Patient ....
Therapist ....

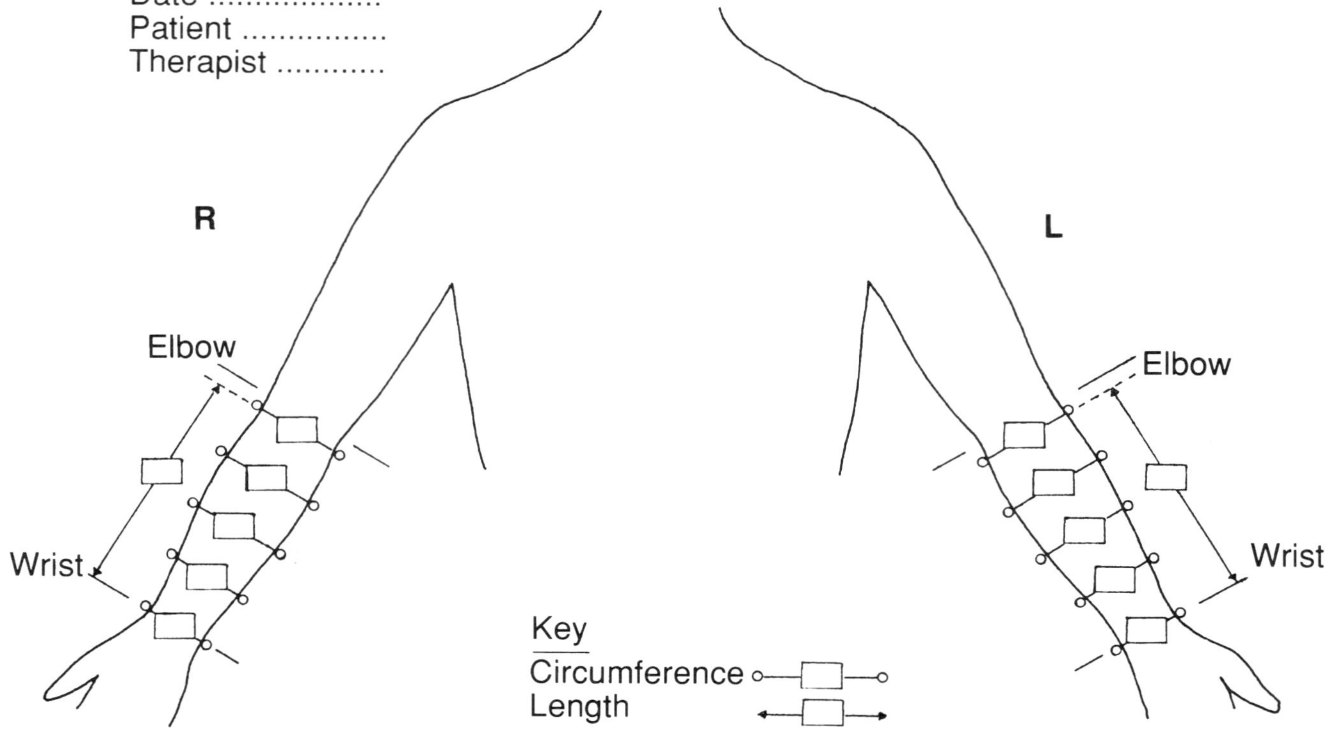

R

L

Elbow

Wrist

Elbow

Wrist

Key
Circumference
Length

4

Torso garments

Before making any garments, please read the general directions in Chapter 2. The garments described in this chapter are:

> **Jacket**
> **Half vest**

JACKET

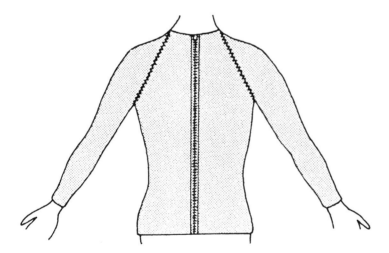

1. Measurements

1a. To make a jacket, use measuring chart number 2, located at the end of this chapter and in Appendix III.

1b. Two sets of measurements are taken for a jacket, i.e. those for the arm and those for the torso.

You will need to decide immediately whether you are using a *V, round* or a *high neckline*, depending on the scar site. Diagrams of these three options will follow.

1c. **Sleeve measurements**

Measure for the length of the sleeve with the arm extended:

    (i) from the wrist to the elbow crease, and
    (ii) from the elbow crease to mid-axilla.

1d. A third length measurement is taken from mid-axilla to the nearest side of the base of the neck (Figure 4.1).

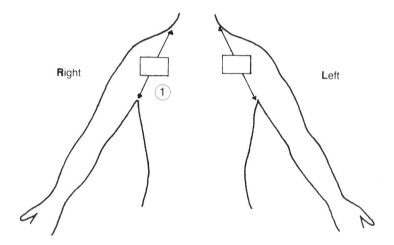

Figure 4.1 **Neck to axilla length measurement**

1e. Next, take the circumferential measurements of each arm at the locations shown on the measuring chart. Generally, these will occur at 5 cm intervals.

1f. **Trunk measurements**

Length measurements are taken:

    (i) from mid-axilla to the greater trochanter of the femur (length line 2)
    (ii) from the middle to the top of the sternum (length line 3), and
    (iii) across the neck, from the base of the lateral aspect of one side to the other (length line 4).

1g. Next, take the circumferential measurements of the torso at the locations shown on the measuring chart. Make a note on the chart of the distance between each of them.

2. Drafting the pattern

2a. Calculate the measurements by:

(i) multiplying all circumferential measurements by 0.4, and

(ii) subtracting 15–20% from each axilla–elbow and elbow–wrist length measurement. Do not alter any other length measurement.

These adjusted measurements are then used to construct your paper pattern. You will need to make three pattern pieces, one for each sleeve and one for the torso.

2b. **Sleeves**

Using a ruler:

(i) Draw a horizontal line on a large piece of blank paper to represent your adjusted wrist–elbow crease and elbow crease–mid-axilla lengths. Mark one end of this line **W**rist and the other **A**xilla. Also mark the position of the elbow crease on this line.

(ii) Use your adjusted wrist (circumferential) measurement to draw a straight line up from the horizontal length line. Repeat this for the axilla measurement (Figure 4.2).

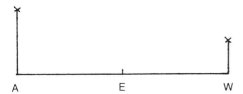

A   E   W

Figure 4.2 **The length, wrist and axilla lines plotted (A, axilla; E, elbow; W, wrist)**

2c. Mark the other adjusted circumferential measurements onto the pattern, ensuring that they are accurately spaced. It is not necessary to draw lines for these measurements, but simply indicate their locations with a small 'x' (Figure 4.3).

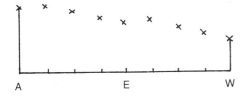

A   E   W

Figure 4.3 **Circumferential arm measurements**

2d. Connect these marks with a pencil line which should flow smoothly to approximate the contours of the arm.

2e. Flare each end of the pattern slightly by no more than 1 cm at the wrist and 1.5 cm at the axilla.

2f. Extend the length line out horizontally from the axilla mark.

2g. Next, take the axilla–neck measurement and subtract 3 cm from it. Use this adjusted length to draw a line down at an angle from the top of the axilla line to join the extended length line. This new line will be referred to as 'length line 1'. These two lines will form a raglan top to the sleeve.

Note. The angle at which these lines meet may have to be altered when fitting the garment. This may involve increasing these length lines so that they meet at a more acute angle. Modifications can be made according to the patient's shape and thus altered on the pattern. Greater accuracy in drafting sleeve tops will come with experience.

Mark the horizontal length line with a 'fold' symbol. This completes the sleeve pattern (Figure 4.4). Cut it out carefully.

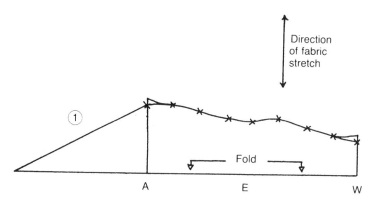

Figure 4.4 **Sleeve pattern**

2h. Torso pattern

Using the axilla–greater trochanter length line, draw a vertical line onto a large blank piece of paper with a ruler.

2i. Mark this line **A**xilla (at the top end) and **B**aseline (for the midpoint between the greater trochanters). This will be referred to as 'length line 2'.

2j. In this pattern, the adjusted circumferential measurements are plotted horizontally so that they are bisected by the vertical length line. This can be achieved by dividing each adjusted circumferential measurement in half. Plot one half on each side of the length line, ensuring that they are accurately spaced. Connect the measurements at the bottom with a straight line to form the bottom edge of the pattern. The other measurements are plotted with an 'x' on either side of the length line (Figure 4.5).

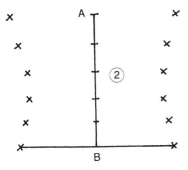

Figure 4.5 **Torso measurements (A, axilla; B, baseline)**

2k. Join the 'x' marks together with a smooth line to approximate the contours of the torso. Flare the pattern at each axilla and at each end of the torso by no more than 1.5 cm.

2l. Add the mid-sternum–top of sternum length line to the top end of length line 2. Mark the sternal end of this line **T**op and label this extension 'length line 3'.

   (i) Adjust the neck length line by subtracting 10 cm from it. This line may need to be altered both in length and position to ensure a close fit around the neck. Accuracy will come with experience.

   (ii) Using this adjusted length, draw a horizontal line approximately 2 cm above the top of the vertical length line so that there is an equal distance on either side of the vertical line. This is referred to as 'length line 4' (Figure 4.6).

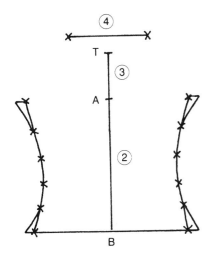

Figure 4.6 **Length lines plotted (T, top)**

2m. Measure the length of the raglan or diagonal edge of each sleeve top (length line 1). Use this length to draw a corresponding line between the appropriate end of length line 4 and the top outer circumferential torso measurements. Some adjustment may be needed to the position of length line 4 to accommodate the length of the raglan sleeve top edge (Figure 4.7).

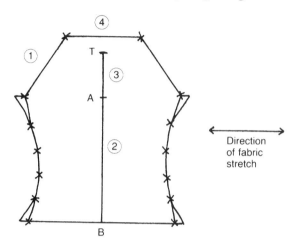

Figure 4.7 **Sleeve insertions**

2n. **Neckline**

For a curved neckline, shape length line 4 to accommodate the anterior neck curve. For a V-neck, draw a dotted line from each end of length line 4 to the top end-point of length line 3. This line will be cut from the front piece of the fabric only. This completes the pattern (Figure 4.8). Cut it out carefully.

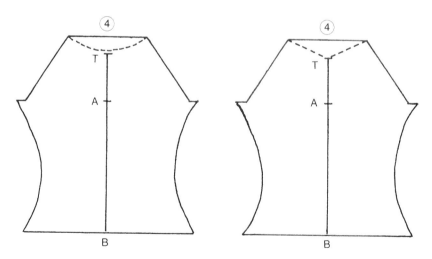

Figure 4.8 **Curved and V-neck outlines**

3. Cutting the fabric

3a. **Sleeves**

Pin the sleeve pattern onto a folded piece of fabric:

(i) ensure that the length line matches the fold of the fabric, and
(ii) that the direction of stretch of the fabric corresponds with the direction of the circumferential measurements and not with the length.

Cut the fabric out, following pattern lines accurately. Mark the fabric **R**ight or **L**eft.

3b. **Torso**

Pin the pattern onto a doubled piece of fabric, ensuring that the direction of stretch corresponds with the circumferential torso measurements and not with the length.

3c. Cut the fabric out following the pattern lines accurately. Mark one piece **F**ront and the other **B**ack.

3d. For a V-neck, mark the top piece of fabric to indicate the neck outline. Once the pattern is removed, cut this outline from the front piece of the fabric only.

4. Sewing the garment

4a. Measure the length of the front torso fabric piece from mid-neck-line to mid-baseline to determine the zipper length required. Centre and insert an open-ended zipper to the right side of the front torso piece of fabric. Cut away the fabric underneath the zipper and insert a backing strip (see Chapter 2).

4b. To insert a sleeve, match length line 1 of the raglan sleeve top to the corresponding length line 1 of the front torso piece. Overlap these length lines by 0.5 cm and join with a flat seam (Figure 4.9).

4c. Repeat this step with the back torso piece.

4d. Repeat steps 4b and 4c for the second sleeve.

4e. With the wrong sides together, pin the inside edges of each sleeve and the torso side seams.

4f. Sew these together with a single zigzag seam of 0.5 cm width, starting at the wrist, continuing around the axilla and down the torso side seam to the end of the garment.

4g. Repeat with the remaining side seam.

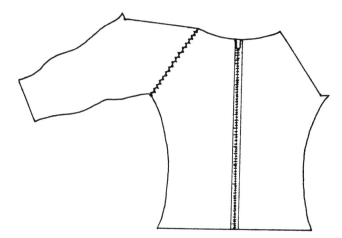

Figure 4.9 **Joining sleeve to torso**

4h. To insert a piece of elastic. Open the jacket and measure the length of the entire bottom edge. Cut a piece of soft elastic (as described in Chapter 2) and sew into place along the inside bottom edge of the jacket, using a long zigzag stitch. This completes the garment (Figure 4.10).

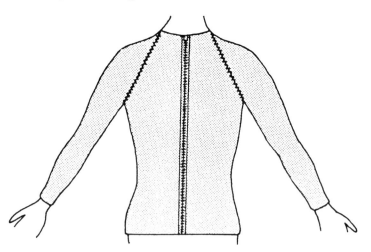

Figure 4.10 **The completed jacket**

5. Fitting the garment

5a. With adult female patients, allowance must be made for the breasts. This can be done by having the patient don her garment at the initial fitting and marking the position of the nipple directly onto the fabric. The patient removes her garment and a hole approximately 5 cm in diameter is cut out around the nipple mark. The garment is refitted and further material cut away as appropriate for comfort, depending on breast size. A small hem

can be made around the edge of the outline to prevent fraying.
The patient can then use her bra over the jacket. The breast outline should be marked onto the paper pattern for future use.

6. Modifications

6a. **Sleeve lengths**

It is always necessary to insert two sleeves into a jacket to achieve
consistent pressure. However, it may not be necessary to have
two full-length sleeves, depending on the site of the scarring.
Shorter sleeves are made by taking the circumferential arm measurements needed along the required sleeve length line. The
raglan top is needed for all sleeves and is made in the way
described earlier.

6b. **Collars**

When scarring is present in or on the neck, it may be helpful to
insert a collar into the neckline of the jacket to apply pressure to
the area. In this case the jacket should be fastened with a zipper
inserted into the middle of the back so that the jacket will open
from the rear. The jacket is designed with a high, round (mandarin
style) collar (Figure 4.11). A strip of Lycra, twice the width of the
desired collar height and the same length as the neckline plus 5
cm for an overlap, is cut out. The collar is fastened with Velcro
sewn into each end. It is essential that the neckline of the jacket
fits very accurately into the base of the neck to ensure consistent
pressure over the neck and chest.

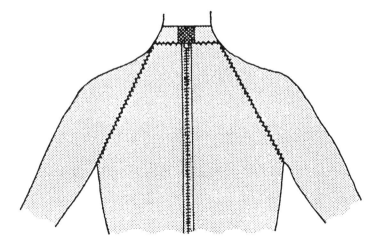

Figure 4.11 **High neck collar (posterior view)**

6c. Elastic (2.5 cm width) can be inserted around the inside neckline of the jacket when a closer fit is required.

6d. **Back-fastening jacket**

A zipper is inserted into the right side of the back torso piece of fabric so that the jacket opens from the rear. Where the patient finds this location of zipper uncomfortable, Velcro can be used instead. This may be indicated where a child consistently undoes a zipper or where better pressure could be applied to a scar site with the zipper relocated.

HALF VEST

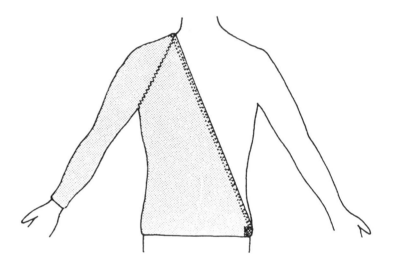

1. Measurements

1a. To make the half vest, use measuring chart number 2 located at the end of this chapter and in Appendix III.

1b. Two sets of measurements are taken:

 (i) those for the arm, and
 (ii) those for the trunk.

1c. **Sleeve measurements**

Measure for the length of the sleeve with the arm extended:

 (i) from the wrist to the elbow crease, and
 (ii) from the elbow crease to mid-axilla.

1d. A third length measurement is taken from mid-axilla to the lateral side of the base of the neck (Figure 4.12).

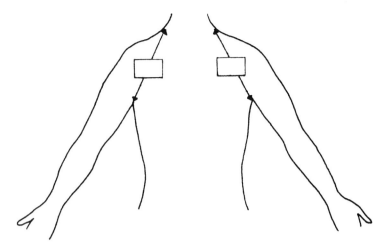

Figure 4.12   **Neck to axilla length measurements**

1e. Next, take the circumferential measurements of the arm at the locations shown on the measuring chart. Generally, these will occur at 5 cm intervals.

1f. **Trunk measurements**

Only two measurements are needed of the trunk for the half vest:

(i) length – from mid-axilla to waist, and
(ii) circumferential – waistline.

2.   Drafting the pattern

2a. Calculate the measurements by

(i) multiplying all the circumferential measurements by 0.4, and
(ii) subtracting 15–20% from each sleeve length measurement. The mid-axilla to waist length remains unchanged.

These adjusted measurements are then used to construct your paper pattern. You will need to make two pattern pieces, one for the sleeve and one for the torso.

2b. **Sleeves**

Using a ruler:

(i) Draw a horizontal line on a large piece of blank paper to represent your adjusted wrist–elbow crease and elbow crease–mid-axilla lengths. Mark one end of this line **W**rist and the other **A**xilla. Also mark the position of the **E**lbow crease on this line.

(ii) Use your adjusted wrist (circumferential) measurement to draw a straight line up from the horizontal length line. Repeat this for the axilla measurement (Figure 4.13).

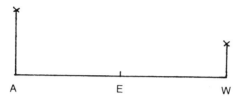

Figure 4.13 **The length, wrist and axilla lines plotted (A, axilla; E, elbow; W, wrist)**

2c. Mark the other adjusted circumferential measurements onto the pattern, ensuring that they are accurately spaced. It is not necessary to draw lines for these measurements; simply indicate their locations with a small 'x' (Figure 4.14).

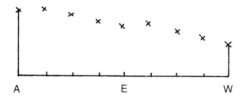

Figure 4.14 **Circumferential arm measurements**

2d. Connect these marks with a pencil line which should flow smoothly to approximate the contours of the arm.

2d. Flare each end of the pattern slightly by no more than 1 cm at the wrist and 1.5 cm at the axilla.

2f. Extend the length line out horizontally from the axilla mark.

2g. Next, take the axilla–neck measurement and subtract 3 cm from it. Use this adjusted length to draw a line down at an angle from the top of the axilla line to join the extended length line. This new line will be referred to as 'length line 1'. These two lines will form a raglan top to the sleeve.

Note. The angle at which these lines meet may have to be altered when fitting the garment. This may involve increasing these length lines so that they meet at a more acute angle. Modifications can be made according to the patient's shape and thus altered on the pattern. Greater accuracy in drafting sleeve tops will come with experience.

Mark the horizontal length line with a 'fold' symbol. This completes the sleeve pattern (Figure 4.15). Cut it out carefully.

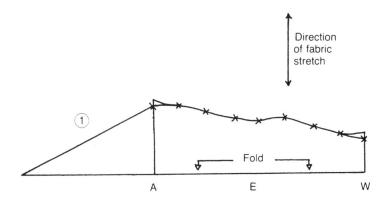

Figure 4.15 **Sleeve pattern completed**

2h. **Torso**

Using the mid-axilla–waist length, draw a vertical line, with a ruler, onto a large blank piece of paper. Mark one end of this line **A**xilla, and the bottom end **W**aist.

2i. Draw a horizontal line out from point W using the adjusted circumferential waist measurement. Mark the end of this line **Z**.

2j. Measure length line 1 (the diagonal measurement) of the sleeve top, and draw a similar line from point A, at an approximate angle of 45°. Mark the end of this line **N**eck (Figure 4.16).

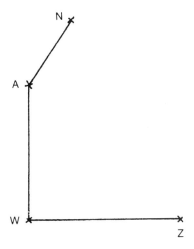

Figure 4.16 **Torso length lines (N, neck; A, axilla; W, waist; Z, adjusted waist measurement)**

2k. Using a ruler, join point N to point Z.

21. Extend the horizontal waist line at point Z by 5 cm. Square this off with dotted lines to form a tab for the garment fastening. This completes the pattern (Figure 4.17). Cut it out carefully.

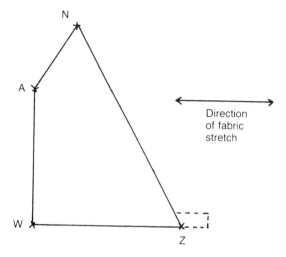

Figure 4.17 **Completed torso pattern**

3. Cutting the fabric

3a. Sleeves

Pin the sleeve pattern onto a folded piece of fabric:

(i) ensure that the length line matches the fold of the fabric, and
(ii) that the direction of stretch of the fabric corresponds with the direction of the circumferential measurements and not with the length.

Cut the pattern out following the pattern lines carefully.

3b. Torso

Pin the pattern onto a doubled piece of fabric. Ensure that the direction of stretch of the fabric corresponds with the direction of the circumferential measurements and not with the length. Cut the pattern out following the pattern lines carefully. Mark one piece of the fabric **Front** and the other **Back**.

3c. The tab is only needed on the back so trim it off the front piece.

4. Sewing the garment

4a. To attach the sleeve, match length line 1 of the sleeve and front torso piece. Overlap them by 0.3 cm and join with a flat seam (Figure 4.18).

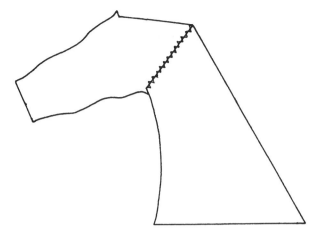

Figure 4.18 **Sewing the sleeve to the torso**

4b. Repeat this step with the back torso piece.

4c. With wrong sides together, pin the inside sleeve and the torso side seam.

4d. Sew these together with a single zigzag seam of 0.5 cm width. Start at the wrist, continue around the axilla and down the torso side seam to the waist.

4e. For a good fit, elastic is inserted around the entire torso opening of the half vest. Measure the length of this opening, from the front of the waistline, over the shoulder and down to the back of the waistline (excluding the tab). Cut a piece of soft elastic (as described in Chapter 2) and sew into place at the inside edge of the opening with a long zigzag stitch.

4f. To prevent the garment slipping at the shoulder, exert a slight tension on the elastic when sewing it into place. To do this, pull the elastic slightly when sewing, from 10 cm before and after reaching the shoulder top. The fabric underneath should not be pulled. In this way a curve is incorporated into the garment.

4g. Sew a piece of soft (loop) Velcro to the inside of the tab, and a piece of hard (hook) Velcro onto the front of the garment to match it. Alternatively, hook and eye fastenings can be used to secure the garment, depending on patient preference.

5. Fitting the garment

5a. With adult female patients, allowance must be made for the breasts. This can be done by having the patient don her garment at the initial fitting and marking a curve for the breast directly onto the fabric. The patient removes her garment and the marked curve is cut out. The patient can then use her bra over or under the vest. The breast curve should be marked onto the pattern for future use. This completes the garment (Figure 4.19).

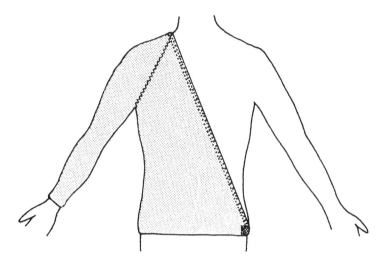

Figure 4.19 **Completed half vest**

Chart No 2: Jacket

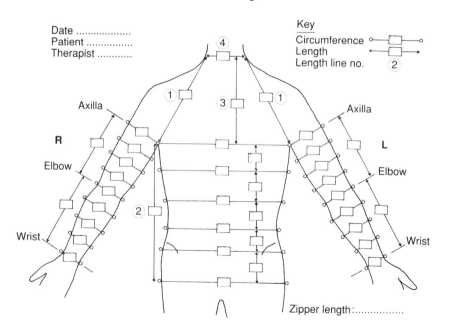

5

Lower limb garments

Please read Chapter 2 before attempting any garments. Those described in this chapter include:

> **Single legging**
> **Double legging**
> **Shorts**
> **Socks**

SINGLE LEGGING

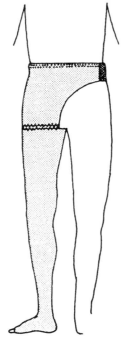

Anterior view

1. Measurements

1a. To make the single legging, use measuring chart number 3 at the end of the chapter and in Appendix III. This garment is made from leg and lower torso measurements in two sections which are then sewn together.

1b. Measure for the length of this garment with the leg in extension. The patient should be standing, if possible. Length measurements are taken from:

   (i) the waist to the buttock crease
   (ii) the buttock crease to the knee
   (iii) the knee to the ankle
   (iv) the ankle to the heel
   (v) the heel to the metatarsal joint of the great toe, and
   (vi) the waist to the heel.

This last measurement is taken to obtain an overall garment length. It can be used to verify the accuracy of the segmental length measurements.

1c. Next, take the circumferential measurements of the leg and foot at the locations shown on the measuring chart. Generally, these will occur at 6 cm intervals.

1d. Take the circumferential measurement of the waist. It is not usually necessary to take any other pelvic measurements

2. Drafting the pattern

2a. Calculate the measurements by:

   (i) multiplying all circumferential measurements by 0.4, and
   (ii) subtracting 15–20% from each length measurement.

These adjusted measurements are then used to construct your paper pattern. Please note that the waist measurement should not be adjusted for this garment.

2b. **Leg pattern**

Using a ruler:

   (i) Draw a single horizontal line on a large piece of blank paper to represent the adjusted buttock crease–knee, knee–ankle, ankle–heel, heel–toe lengths. Mark one end of this line **T**oe and the other **B**uttock. Also mark the position of the **K**nee, **A**nkle and **H**eel on this line.

(ii) Use your adjusted buttock crease circumferential measurement to draw a vertical line up from the horizontal length line. Repeat this for the toe measurement (Figure 5.1).

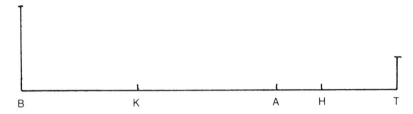

Figure 5.1 **Leg length, buttock and toe measurements (B, buttock; K, knee; A, ankle; H, heel; T, toe)**

2c. Mark the other adjusted circumferential measurements onto the pattern, ensuring that they are accurately spaced. It is not necessary to draw lines for these measurements; simply indicate their locations with a small 'x' (Figure 5.2).

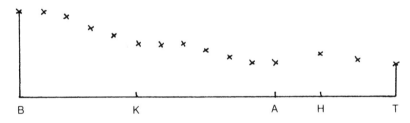

Figure 5.2 **Circumferential leg measurements**

2d. Connect these marks with a pencil line which should approximate the contours of the leg and foot.

2e. Flare each end of the pattern slightly by no more than 1 cm at the toe and 2 cm at the buttock crease. Mark the horizontal line with a fold symbol.

2f. To ensure a good fit at the ankle, a heel dart will have to be made. Take one-third of the adjusted heel circumferential measurement, and mark this point with an 'x', measuring up from the horizontal line at the heel. Draw two lines down from this point to approximately 2 cm either side of the heel. Cut this "V" shape out (Figure 5.3). This completes the leg pattern (Figure 5.4). Cut it out carefully.

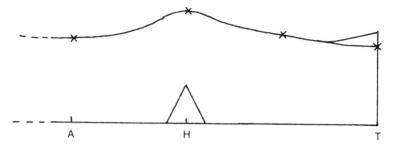

Figure 5.3 **Heel dart**

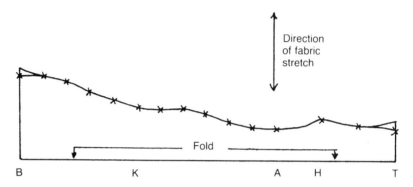

Figure 5.4 **Completed pattern**

2g. **Lower torso pattern**
Using a ruler:

(i) Draw a single horizontal line on a piece of blank paper to represent the adjusted waist–buttock crease length measurement. Mark one end of this line **W**aist and the other **B**uttock.

(ii) Measure the buttock crease line on the leg pattern, subtract 20%, and use this new measurement to draw a vertical line up at the buttock end of the horizontal line.

(iii) Take half the circumferential waist measurement and use this length to draw a vertical line up from the waist end of the horizontal line (Figure 5.5).

2h. Draw a horizontal line out from the end of the waist circumferential line, approximately 5 cm long. This will form the waist band.

For the overweight patient, this line will need to be extended further up to prevent the waist band from rolling down. If necessary, additional hip circumferential measurements may be taken and included on the pattern to accommodate this problem.

Connect this line at the top of the buttock line with a curve. Mark the waist–buttock line with a fold symbol. This completes the lower torso pattern (Figure 5.6). Cut it out carefully.

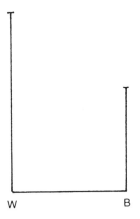

Figure 5.5 **Length and circumferential lines plotted (W, waist; B, buttock)**

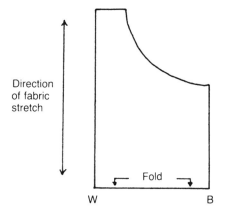

Figure 5.6 **Completed lower torso pattern**

3. Cutting the fabric

3a. Pin both patterns onto a folded piece of Lycra fabric:

   (i) ensure that the length lines match the fold of the fabric, and

   (ii) that the direction of fabric stretch corresponds with the circumferential leg measurements and not the length.

3b. Cut the fabric out, following the pattern lines accurately. Remove the pattern.

4. Sewing the garment

4a. Cut a piece of elastic to match the waist measurement. Sew into place along the inside top edge of the torso piece, using a long zigzag stitch.

4b. Sew a piece of soft (loop) Velcro down one side of the waist band opening, and a piece of hard (hook) Velcro on the other side to match it (Figure 5.7).

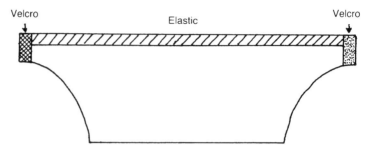

Figure 5.7 **Elastic and Velcro on the torso piece**

4c. Unfold the leg piece. To create the foot dart, fold the leg piece with wrong sides together at the ankle, widthways. This will serve to align the edges of the dart along its length. Pin and sew these edges together with a 0.3 cm seam.

4d. Fold the legging along its length and pin the edges together. Sew into place with a 0.3 cm seam.

4e. To join the torso and leg pieces together, overlap the top of the leg section with the bottom edge of the torso section by 1 cm, so that the leg seam will run down the back of the leg. Pin together. Note that the torso section will be narrower at the top of the leg to accommodate the perineal area. Sew these sections together with a flat double seam to ensure the join is secure (Figure 5.8).

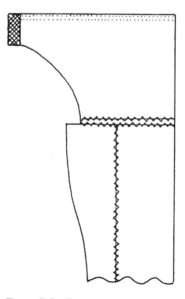

Figure 5.8 **Torso and leg pieces joined: posterior view**

5. Fitting the garment

5a. Accommodation should be made for the peroneal and buttock areas for both patient comfort and hygiene purposes. This can be done by having the patient don the single legging and drawing a line directly onto the fabric. This line should follow a smooth curve between the pelvic side seam and the top of the thigh. Excess fabric is trimmed, and a small 0.5 cm hem sewn around this curve with a long zigzag stitch to prevent fraying. Any alteration to the garment should be noted on the pattern for future reference. This completes the garment (Figure 5.9).

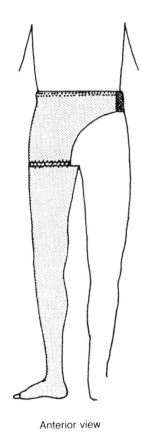

Anterior view

Figure 5.9 **The completed single legging: anterior view**

DOUBLE LEGGING

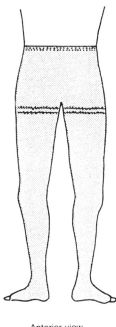

Anterior view

Design note

For *men* with bilateral leg scars, we suggest making two single leggings. This seems to provide maximum comfort and convenience. For *women*, the leg sections can be attached to a pantie-style torso section, similar to pantihose.

1. Measurements

1a. To make the double legging, use measuring chart number 3 at the end of the chapter and in Appendix III.

1b. Measure for the length of this garment with the leg in extension. Ideally the patient should be standing with the ankle at its usual right angle if possible. If your patient is unable to stand, the measurements should be taken with them lying supine. Length measurements are taken from:

   (i) the waist to the buttock crease
   (ii) the buttock crease to the top circumferential measurement of the leg
   (iii) the top circumferential leg measurement to the knee
   (iv) the knee to the ankle
   (v) the ankle to the heel

(vi) the heel to the metatarsal arch of the great toe, and

(vii) the waist to the heel

This last measurement is taken to obtain an overall garment length. It can be used to verify the accuracy of segmental length measurements.

1c. Next, take the circumferential measurements of the leg and foot at the locations shown on the measuring chart. Generally these will occur at 6 cm intervals.

Torso measurements

1d. To make the torso/pantie section, use the same measuring chart.

1e. Measure the following lengths:

(i) waist to buttock crease, and

(ii) buttock crease to top leg circumferential measurement (approximately 5 cm).

1f. Next, take the pelvic circumferential measurements at the locations shown on the measuring chart.

1g. Take the buttock crease circumferential measurement of each leg and the circumferential measurement 5 cm below this (this last measurement should be the same as the top circumferential measurement of the legging).

2. Drafting the pattern

2a. Calculate the measurements by:

(i) multiplying all the circumferential measurements by 0.4, and

(ii) subtracting 15–20% from each length measurement.

These adjusted measurements are then used to construct your paper pattern.

2b. Using a ruler, draw a vertical line at the top end of a large piece of blank paper to represent the adjusted waist–buttock crease length line. Mark the top end **W**aist and the other end **B**uttock.

2c. In this pattern the adjusted circumferential pelvic measurements are plotted horizontally so that they are bisected by the vertical length line. This can be achieved by dividing each adjusted circumferential measurement in half. Plot one half on each side of the length line, using small x's. Ensure that they are accurately spaced.

2d. Using a ruler, connect the two top x's with a straight line to form the top edge of the pattern (Figure 5.10).

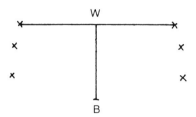

Figure 5.10   **Pelvic measurements (W, waist; B, buttock)**

2e. The length lines for each leg extend from the same point B. They should be drawn with a ruler and separated slightly in order to plot the circumferential measurements of each leg easily.

2f. Using the adjusted length measurement for one leg, draw a line from point B to represent the buttock crease–top of leg length. Mark the end of this line **Leg**. Repeat this step for the opposite leg's adjusted length measurement (Figure 5.11).

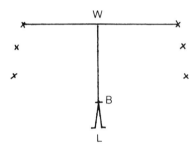

Figure 5.11   **Buttock crease to top of leg measurements (L, leg)**

2g. Use the adjusted top of leg circumferential measurement to draw a straight line out from point L. This will form the bottom edge of the torso or pantie pattern.

2h. Repeat this step for the other leg (Figure 5.12).

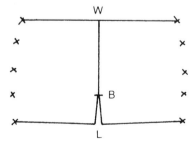

Figure 5.12   **Buttock measurements plotted**

2i. Connect these 'x' marks from the top of the leg to the waist with a pencil line which should flow smoothly to approximate the contours of the body.

2j. Flare the waist by 2 cm at each end of the pattern.

Mark each side of the pattern **R**ight or **L**eft as appropriate. This completes the pattern (Figure 5.13). Cut it out carefully.

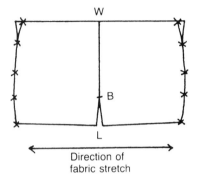

Figure 5.13 **Torso pattern plotted**

2k. **Leg pattern(s)**

Note. You will need to repeat these steps for each leg separately.

Using a ruler:

(i) Draw a single horizontal line on a large piece of blank paper to represent the adjusted top leg circumferential measurement, knee–ankle, ankle–heel, heel–toe lengths. Mark one end of this line **T**oe and the other **B**uttock. Also mark the position of the **K**nee, **A**nkle and **H**eel on this line.

(ii) Use your adjusted top of leg circumferential measurement to draw a vertical line up from the horizontal length line. Repeat this for the toe measurement (Figure 5.14).

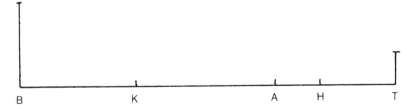

Figure 5.14 **Leg length, buttock and toe measurements (B, buttock; K, knee; A, ankle; H, heel; T, toe)**

2l. Mark the other adjusted circumferential measurements onto the pattern, ensuring that they are accurately spaced. It is not necessary to draw lines for these measurements, simply indicate their locations with a small 'x' (Figure 5.15).

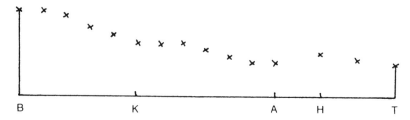

Figure 5.15 **Circumferential leg measurements**

2m. Connect these marks with a pencil line which should approximate the contours of the leg and foot.

2n. Flare each end of the pattern slightly by no more than 1 cm at the toe and 2 cm at the buttock crease. Mark the horizontal line with a fold symbol.

2o. To ensure a good fit at the ankle and heel, a dart will have to be made (Figure 5.16). Take one-third of the adjusted heel circumferential measurement, and mark this point with an 'x', measuring up from the horizontal line at the heel. Draw two lines down from this point to approximately 2 cm either side of the heel. Cut this 'V' shape out. This completes the leg pattern (Figure 5.17). Cut it out carefully.

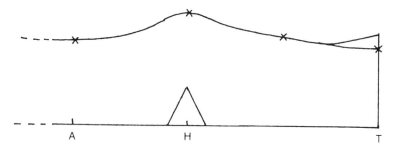

Figure 5.16 **Heel dart**

3. Cutting the fabric

3a. Pin the pantie and leg(s) patterns onto a doubled piece of Lycra fabric, ensuring that the direction of fabric stretch corresponds with the circumferential leg or abdomen measurements, and not with the length.

3b. Cut the fabric, following the pattern lines accurately.

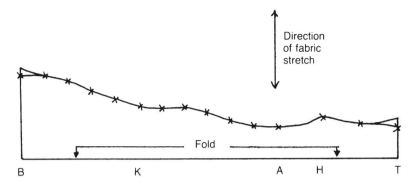

Figure 5.17 **Completed leg(s) pattern**

3c. Remove the pattern. Mark the fabric **F**ront, **B**ack, **L**eft and **R**ight, as appropriate.

4. Sewing the garment

4a. For female patients, a gusset can be inserted into the crotch. Cut a slit 7–8 cm long in both the front and back pieces of the fabric at the point where the torso and leg pieces meet (Figure 5.18).

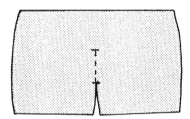

Figure 5.18 **Cutting line for gusset insertion**

4b. To make the gusset, cut a diamond shape out from a single piece of fabric so that one of the long points of the gusset overlaps by 0.5 cm at the top of the slit. Overlap and pin the two corresponding long edges of the gusset with the edges of the slit. Sew this piece into place with a flat double seam to ensure a strong join (Figure 5.19). Repeat this for the back piece with the remaining gusset edges.

4c. With wrong sides together, pin and sew both inside leg seams of the pantie with a double seam. Remember to keep your seams to a 0.3 cm width.

4d. Pin and sew one of the outer leg edges with a double seam.

4e. Unfold the fabric and measure the length of the waistline. Cut a piece of soft elastic (as described in Chapter 2) and sew into place along the inside edge of the waist using a long zigzag stitch.

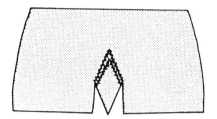

Figure 5.19 **Inserting the gusset**

4f. Unfold one leg piece. To create the foot dart, fold the leg piece with wrong sides together at the ankle, widthways. This will serve to align the edges of the dart along its length. Pin and sew these edges together with a 0.3 cm seam. Repeat for the other leg.

4g. Fold one leg piece along its length and pin the edges together. Sew into place with a 0.3 cm seam. Repeat for the other leg.

4h. To join the torso and leg pieces together, overlap the top of the leg section with the bottom edge of the torso section by 1 cm, so that the leg seam will run down the back of the leg. Pin together. Sew these sections together with a flat double seam to ensure the join is secure (Figure 5.20).

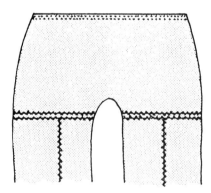

Figure 5.20 **Leg and torso pieces joined: posterior view**

5. Fitting the garment

5a. It will probably be necessary to cut a keyhole shape around the perineum, particularly for male patients. This can be achieved by having the patient don his leggings and drawing a line directly onto the fabric. Excess fabric is cut away and a small 0.5 cm hem is sewn around this opening with a long zigzag stitch to prevent fraying.

5b. This alteration is also helpful for:

    (i) all patients who have difficulty donning garments

    (ii) maintaining good hygiene, and

    (iii) patient comfort.

The patient's preference should be established. Any alteration to the garment should be noted on the pattern for future reference. This completes the garment (Figure 5.21).

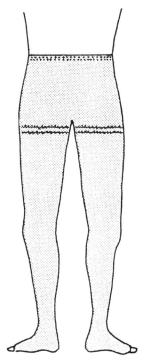

Figure 5.21 **Completed double leggings: anterior view**

6. Modifications

6a. **Leg lengths**

It is not always necessary to make this garment with two full-length legs. Simply amend the length lines and the number of circumferential measurements accordingly.

6b. **Zippers**

Occasionally patients may have difficulty donning this garment, particularly in the early stages when they are unused to pressure therapy. Zippers can be inserted into the garment, approximately mid-calf, to make donning easier. They are inserted first, with backing strips, before any side seams are sewn (Figure 5.22).

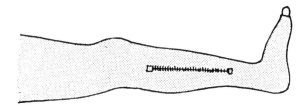

Figure 5.22 **Zipper insertion, mid-calf: lateral view**

SHORTS

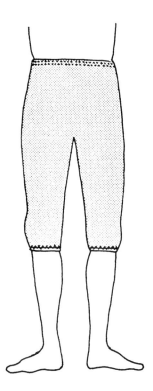

1. Measurements

1a. To make shorts, use measuring chart number 3 at the end of this chapter and in Appendix III.

1b. To take the measurements required for this garment, the legs should be extended and the patient standing, where possible. For patient comfort, shorts usually extend to just below the knees, i.e. by approximately 10 cm.

1c. Measure the following lengths:

   (i) waist to buttock crease, and
   (ii) buttock crease to knee.

1d. Next, take the circumferential measurements of each leg at the locations shown on the measuring chart. Remember to add one or two below the knees. Generally your measurements will occur at 6 cm intervals.

1e. Take the circumferential measurements of the pelvis at the locations shown on the measuring chart. Make a note on the chart of the distances between each of them.

2. Drafting the pattern

2a. Calculate the measurements by:

   (i) multiplying all circumferential measurements by 0.4, and
   (ii) subtracting 15–20% from each length measurement.

   These adjusted measurements are used to construct your paper pattern. *Note*: If the pelvis is not scarred, pelvic circumferential measurements do not have to be adjusted.

2b. Using a ruler, draw a vertical line at the top end of a large piece of blank paper to represent the adjusted waist–buttock crease length line. Mark the top end **W**aist and the other end **B**uttock.

2c. In this pattern the adjusted circumferential pelvic measurements are plotted horizontally so that they are bisected by the vertical length line. This can be achieved by dividing each adjusted circumferential measurement in half. Plot one half on each side of the length line, using small x's. Ensure that they are accurately spaced.

2d. Using a ruler, connect the two top x's with a straight line to form the top edge of the pattern (Figure 5.23).

2e. The length lines for each leg extend from the same point B. They should be drawn with a ruler and separated slightly in order to plot the circumferential measurements of each leg easily.

2f. Using the adjusted length measurements for one leg, draw a line from point B to represent the buttock crease–knee joint length. Continue this line by adding the adjusted knee joint–below-knee length. Mark these positions **K** and **B/K** on this line. Repeat this step for the opposite leg's adjusted length measurements (Figure 5.24).

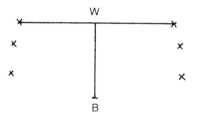

Figure 5.23 **Pelvic measurements (W, waist; B, buttock)**

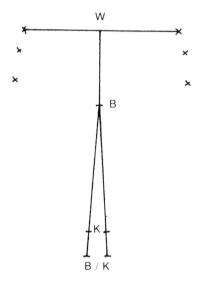

Figure 5.24 **Leg length measurements (K, knee; B/K, below knee)**

2g. Use the adjusted below-knee circumferential measurement to draw a straight line out from point B/K. This will form the bottom edge of the leg's pattern.

2h. Mark the other adjusted circumferential measurements onto the pattern, ensuring that they are accurately spaced. It is not necessary to draw lines for these measurements; simply indicate their locations with small x's. Repeat this step for the other leg (Figure 5.25).

2i. Connect these 'x' marks from the waist to the end of the B/K circumferential line with a pencil line which should flow smoothly to approximate the contours of the body.

2j. Flare each end of the pattern slightly:

    (i) by no more than 1.5 cm below each knee, and
    (ii) by no more than 2 cm on each side of the waist line.

Mark each leg **Left** or **Right** as appropriate. This completes the pattern (Figure 5.26). Cut it out carefully.

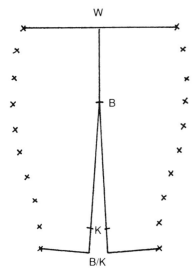

Figure 5.25 **Circumferential leg measurements**

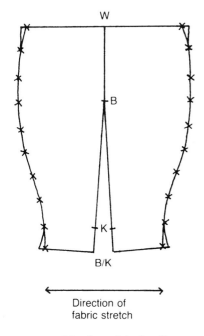

Direction of
fabric stretch

Figure 5.26 **Completed pattern**

3. Cutting the fabric

3a. Pin the pattern onto a doubled piece of Lycra fabric, ensuring that
the direction of fabric stretch corresponds with the circumferential
leg measurements, and not with the length.

3b. Cut the fabric, following the pattern lines accurately.

3c. Remove the pattern. Mark the fabric **F**ront and **B**ack as appropriate.

4. Sewing the garment

4a. For female patients a gusset can be inserted into the crotch. Cut a slit 7–8 cm long in both the front and back pieces of fabric, from the point where the two legs meet up into the body (Figure 5.27).

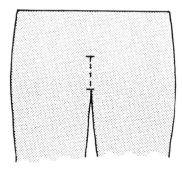

Figure 5.27   **Cutting line for gusset insertion**

4b. To make the gusset, cut a diamond shape out from a single piece of fabric so that one of the long points of the gusset overlaps by 0.5 cm at the top of the slit. Overlap and pin the two corresponding long edges of the gusset with the edges of the slit. Sew this into place with a flat double seam to ensure a strong join. Repeat this for the back piece with the two remaining gusset edges (Figure 5.28).

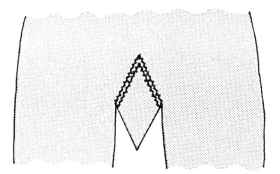

Figure 5.28   **Inserting the gusset**

4c. With wrong sides together, pin and sew both inside leg seams with a double seam. Remember to keep your seams to a 0.3 cm width.

4d. Sew a hem approximately 2–3 cm wide along the bottom edge of each leg using a long zigzag stitch. This will prevent the garment from rolling up.

4e. Pin and sew with one side of the outer legs with a double seam.

4f. Unfold the fabric and measure the length of the waistline. Cut a piece of soft elastic and sew into place along the inside edge of the waist using a long zigzag stitch.

4g. With wrong sides together, pin and sew the second outside leg seam.

5. Fitting the garment

5a. It will probably be necessary to cut a keyhole shape around the perineum, particularly for male patients. This can be achieved by having the patient don the shorts and drawing a line directly onto the fabric. Excess fabric is cut away and a small 0.5 cm hem is sewn around this opening with a long zigzag stitch to prevent fraying (Figure 5.29). Any alteration to the garment should be noted on the pattern for future reference.

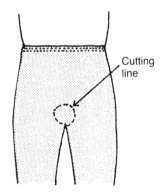

Cutting line

Figure 5.29 **Keyhole opening in shorts: anterior view**

5b. This alteration is also helpful for:

    (i) all patients who have difficulty donning garments
    (ii) maintaining personal hygiene, and
    (iii) patient comfort.

The patient's preference should be established. This completes the garment (Figure 5.30).

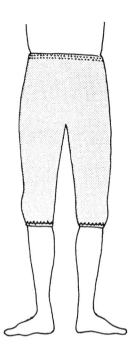

Figure 5.30 **Completed shorts**

6. Modifications

6a. It is not always necessary to make this garment extend below the knee. Simply amend the length lines and the number of circumferential measurements accordingly.

BELOW-KNEE SOCK

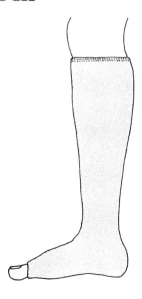

1. Measurements

1a. To make the below-knee sock use measuring chart 4 at the end of the chapter and in Appendix III.

1b. Measure for the length of this garment with the leg in extension and the patient standing, if possible.

Length measurements are taken from:

(i) just below the knee to the ankle
(ii) ankle to heel, and
(iii) heel to metatarsal joint of the great toe.

1c. Next, take the circumferential measurements of the leg and foot at the locations shown on the measuring chart. Generally, these will occur at 5 cm intervals.

2. Drafting the pattern

2a. Calculate the measurements by:

(i) multiplying all circumferential measurements by 0.4, and
(ii) subtracting 15–20% from each leg and foot length measurement.

These adjusted measurements are then used to construct the paper pattern.

2b. Using a ruler:

(i) Draw a single horizontal line onto a piece of blank paper to represent the adjusted knee–ankle, ankle–heel and heel–toe lengths. Mark one end of this line **K**nee and the other **T**oe. Also mark the position of the ankle and heel.
(ii) Use your adjusted circumferential knee measurement to draw a vertical line up from the horizontal length line at the knee end. Repeat this for the toe measurement (Figure 5.31).

2c. Mark the other adjusted circumferential measurements onto the pattern, ensuring that they are accurately spaced. It is not necessary to draw lines for these measurements; simply indicate their locations with a small 'x' (Figure 5.32).

2d. Connect these measurements with a pencil line which should flow smoothly to approximate the contours of the leg and foot.

2e. Flare each end of the pattern slightly by no more than 1 cm at the toe and 1.5 cm at the knee. Mark the horizontal line with a fold symbol (Figure 5.33).

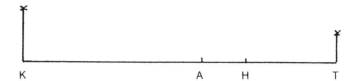

Figure 5.31 **Length, knee and toe lines plotted (K, knee; A, ankle; H, heel; T, toe)**

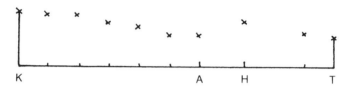

Figure 5.32 **Circumferential measurements plotted**

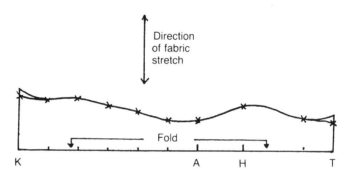

Figure 5.33 **Flared pattern**

2f. To achieve a good fit at the ankle and heel, a dart will have to be made. Take one-third of the adjusted circumferential heel measurement and mark this point with an 'x', measuring up for the horizontal line at the heel. Draw two lines down from this point to approximately 2 cm on either side of the heel. Cut this 'V' shape out (Figure 5.34). This completes the sock pattern. Cut it out carefully.

3. Cutting the fabric

3a. Pin the pattern onto a folded piece of Lycra fabric, ensuring that the:

    (i) length line matches the fold of the fabric, and
    (ii) direction of fabric stretch corresponds with the circumferential calf measurements and not the length.

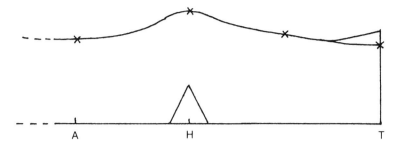

A   H   T

Figure 5.34 **Heel dart**

3b. Cut the fabric out, including the darts, following the pattern lines accurately. Remove the pattern.

4. Sewing the garment

4a. Unfold the fabric. Cut a piece of soft elastic 1 cm longer than the width of the garment at its knee end. This will give you 0.5 cm excess at either edge.

4b. Sew into place along the inside edge of the sock top using a long zigzag stitch.

4c. To sew the foot dart, fold the leg piece with wrong sides together at the ankle across its width. This will align the edges of the dart along its length. Pin and sew these edges together with a 0.3 cm seam.

4d. Fold the sock along its length and pin the edges together. Join them with a 0.3 cm seam. Trim excess elastic to finish.

5. Fitting the garment

5a. Owing to the curve of the heel, this seam may need to be altered once fitted on the patient. Note any changes made to the garment onto the pattern.

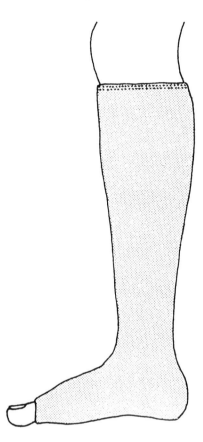

Figure 5.35 **Completed sock**

6. Modifications

6a. When scarring extends to the toes, the sock should be extended to accommodate the toe length. In severe cases, trace the outline of the toes directly onto the fabric with a pen and sew around this outline to close the end of the sock. This will provide more consistent pressure to the area.

6b. **Above-knee sock**

The length of the sock can be extended as required, by taking additional length and circumferential measurements.

Chart No. 3: Leggings/shorts

Date ....
Patient ....
Therapist ....

Key
Circumference
Length

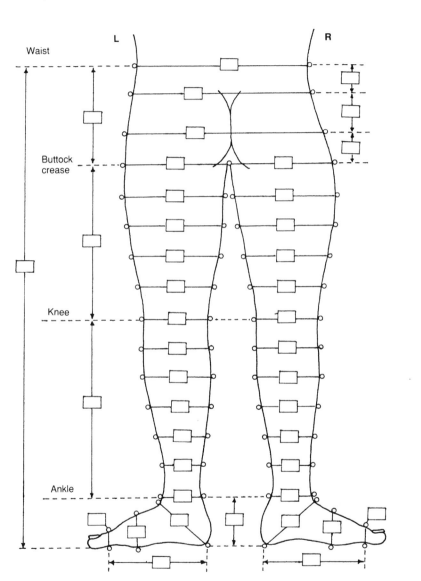

Waist

Buttock crease

Knee

Ankle

L   R

Chart No. 4: Below-knee sock

Date ....
Patient ....
Therapist ....

Key

Circumference

Length

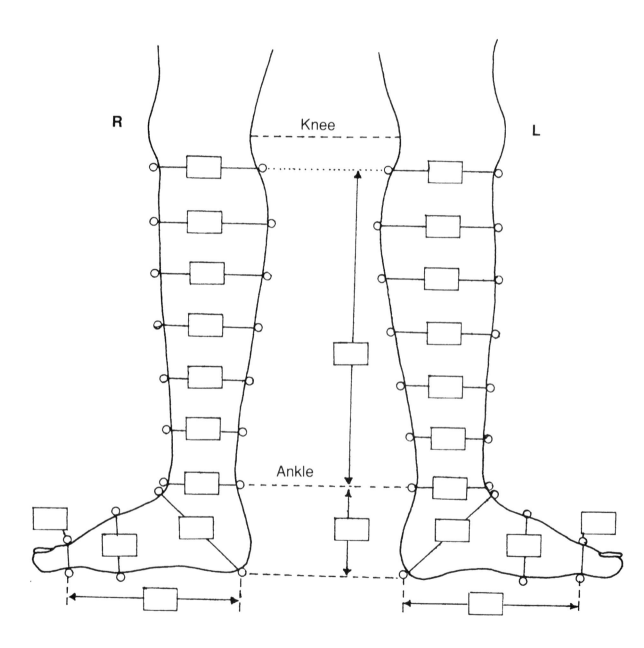

R   Knee   L

Ankle

6

Head garments

Please read the general instructions in Chapter 2 before making any of the garments. This chapter will include directions for the:

> **Mask**
>
> **Chin strap**

FULL MASK

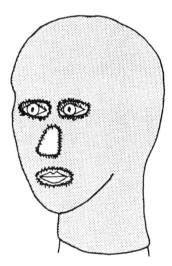

This garment is one of the most difficult to make. Much of the pattern can only be completed after an initial fitting on the patient.

1. Measurements

1a. To make a mask use measuring chart number 5 at the end of the chapter and in Appendix III.

1b. Measure for the lengths needed in the mask from:

    (i) the top of the head, over the ear, to the base of the neck (lateral aspect)
    (ii) mid-forehead to the point of the chin, and
    (iii) the point of the chin to the anterior base of the neck.

1c. Circumferential measurements of the head are needed around the:

    (i) mid-forehead (designated **A**)
    (ii) eyes/bridge of nose (**B**)
    (iii) mouth (**C**)
    (iv) neck at two locations, and
    (v) base of the neck (**D**).

Note the distance between each of these on the measuring chart.

2. Drafting the pattern

2a. Calculate the measurements needed by dividing each circumferential measurement in half. No further adjustments are made to the length or circumferential measurements until the garment is fitted.

2b. Using a ruler, draw a vertical line onto a blank piece of paper to represent the head–neck length measurement.

2c. Using the halved circumferential measurements (A, B, C and D) draw horizontal lines across the length line so that one-third of each measurement is on the right of this line, i.e. in front of the ear, and two-thirds on the left of it, i.e. at the back of the ear. Mark the additional neck measurements onto the pattern. Ensure that they are accurately spaced (Figure 6.1).

2d. Join the ends of the circumferential lines from the front end of line A (forehead) to the top of the length line, continuing around the back ends of lines A, B and C, finishing at line D. This line should accommodate each individual patient's skull shape as closely as possible.

2e. Draw the mid-forehead–chin length line down from and at a right angle to the front end of line A. Mark the end of this new line **E** and add a 'fold' symbol to it.

2f. Join point E to the front end of line D with a curve that will accommodate the anterior neck shape.

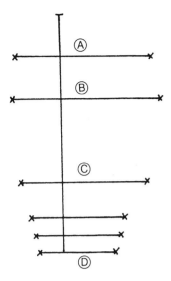

Figure 6.1 **Circumferential measurements (A, mid-forehead; B, eyes/bridge of nose; C, mouth; D, base of the neck)**

2g. Flare the pattern at the neck opening by no more than 2 cm (Figure 6.2). Cut the pattern out carefully.

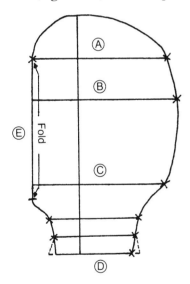

Figure 6.2 **Drafted pattern**

3. Cutting the fabric

3a. Pin the pattern onto a folded piece of fabric:

    (i) ensuring that the 'fold' symbol corresponds with the fold of the fabric, and

(ii) the direction of stretch of the fabric corresponds with the circumferential measurements of the head and not the length.

3b. Cut the fabric out following the pattern lines accurately.

4. Sewing the garment

4a. With wrong sides together, pin and sew the mask from the forehead to the occipital bone (base of skull) only. This will create the opening necessary for donning the garment so that it will fit over the head. Velcro strips are sewn in to ensure a snug fit.

4b. Sew the chin–anterior base of neck seam with a zigzag stitch of 0.5 cm width.

5. Fitting the garment

5a. Have the patient don the garment. Mark the outline of the eyes, nose and mouth.

5b. Remove the mask from the patient and cut these shapes out.

5c. Refit the garment and alter the size of these shapes as necessary. Ensure that the hole over the nose extends to the bridge, for patient comfort. Hem the outline of the holes with a 0.5 cm long zigzag stitch.

5d. Adjust the seams of the garment to achieve consistent pressure and patient comfort. Trim away excess fabric and mark the pattern accordingly.

5e. Add straps or Velcro along the length of the opening at the back of the neck for a good fit. This completes the garment (Figure 6.3).

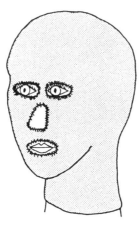

Figure 6.3 **Completed full mask**

6. Modifications

If there is no scarring near the ears, openings can be cut out for them, for patient comfort.

CHIN STRAP

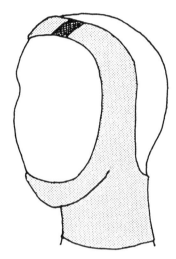

Chin straps can be made using the outlines at the end of the chapter and in Appendix IV, to make a template. This template can then be used to make the pattern for most adults, with only minor adjustments. Simply copy the template, hold it against the patient, and amend the shape where necessary with a pen. Cut away excess pattern or use arrows to indicate on the pattern where it needs to be widened. However, you may find it necessary to draft your own pattern when treating children or small/large adults.

1. Measurements

1a. To make a chin strap, use measuring chart 6 at the end of the chapter and in Appendix III. Using the temporomandibular joint (TMJ) as the centre point, take the following length measurements:

    (i) from the TMJ to the top of the head (**1**)
    (ii) from the TMJ to the chin crease (**2**)
    (iii) from the TMJ to the lateral aspect of the base of the neck (**3**)
    (iv) from the TMJ to the occiput (**4**)
    (v) from the occiput to the posterior base of the neck (**5**), and
    (vi) from the chin crease to the anterior base of the neck (**6**).

2. Drafting the pattern

2a. Use the TMJ as the starting point for your pattern. Make a mark 'x' to indicate its position on a blank piece of paper.

2b. Using a ruler, draw lines from the 'x' to represent length lines 1, 2, 3 and 4. The angles at which these lines are drawn should approximate the patient's profile as closely as possible (Figure 6.4).

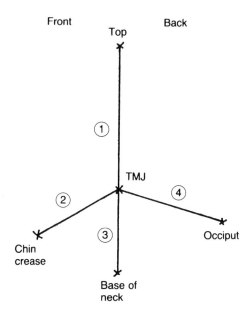

Figure 6.4 **Chin strap lengths plotted (TMJ, temporomandibular joint)**

2c. Draw a line from the end of line 4 to represent the length of line 5.

2d. Draw a line from the end of line 2 to represent length 6.

Both lines 5 and 6 should be drawn to accommodate the width and shape of the chin and neck as closely as possible.

2e. Join the ends of lines 5, 3 and 6 to form the base of the pattern (Figure 6.5).

2f. Draw a horizontal line across the end of line 1 approximately 5 cm wide to represent the top of the garment. Label this new line 7. Join the end of line 4 to the end of line 7 with a curve that will pass behind the ear.

2g. Join the end of line 2 to the end of line 7 with a curve that will pass mid-way between the front of the ear and the eye. This completes the pattern (Figure 6.6). Cut it out carefully.

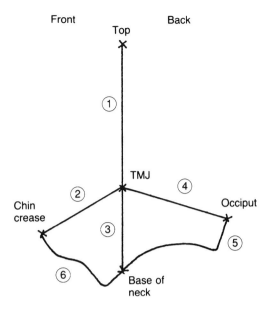

Figure 6.5 **Chin and neck profile**

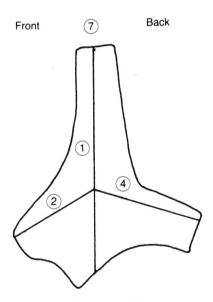

Figure 6.6 **Pattern outline**

3. Cutting the fabric

3a. Pin the pattern onto a doubled piece of fabric, ensuring that the direction of the fabric stretch corresponds with the width of the neck and not the length. Cut the fabric out following the pattern lines accurately.

4. Sewing the garment

4a. Overlap the edges of the pieces of fabric from the chin to the anterior base of the neck by 0.5 cm and sew together with a flat seam.

4b. Sew a piece of soft (loop) Velcro to the inside top of one head strap. Sew a piece of hard (hook) Velcro to match, on the outside of the opposite head strap.

4c. Repeat this step with the opening at the back of the neck.

5. Fitting the garment

5a. Have the patient don the chin strap. It may be necessary to adjust the chin seam or to make darts where there is excess fabric. Mark any alterations made onto the paper pattern for future reference.

5b. Sew a 0.5 cm hem around the facial opening for patient comfort and to prevent fraying.

5c. Repeat this for the opening at the back of the head. This completes the garment (Figure 6.7).

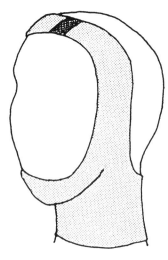

Figure 6.7 **The completed chin strap**

Caution

Mandibular shortening has been noted in children when excessive pressure has been exerted on the chin. It is essential that the amount of pressure exerted on this site is monitored. There is current research evidence to suggest that pressures between 5 and 12 mmHg are sufficient and effective in altering scar configurations. A pressure manometer, described in Chapter 2, which measures interface pressure can be used for this purpose.

Chart No. 5: Full mask

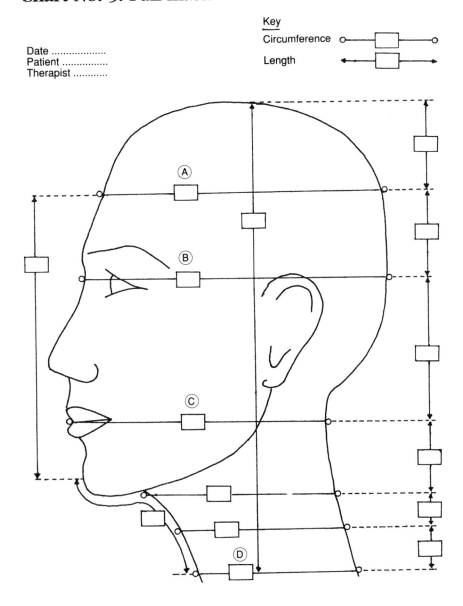

Key
Circumference o———☐———o
Length ◄———☐———►

Date ....
Patient ....
Therapist ....

Chart No. 6: Chin strap

Key
<u>Length</u>

Line no.

Date ....
Patient ....
Therapist ....

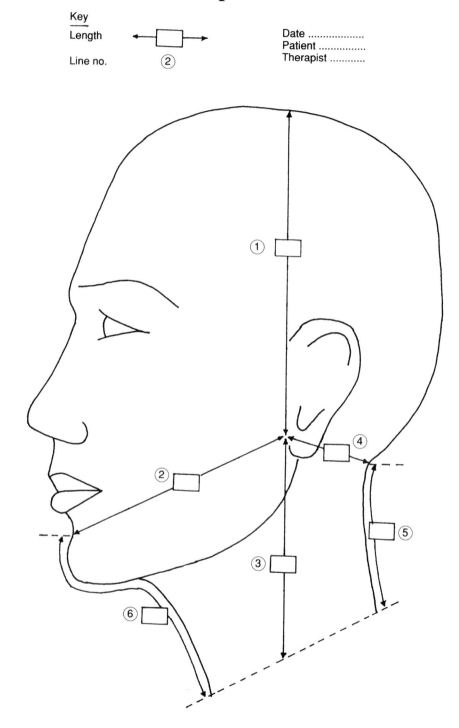

Chin strap 1 template

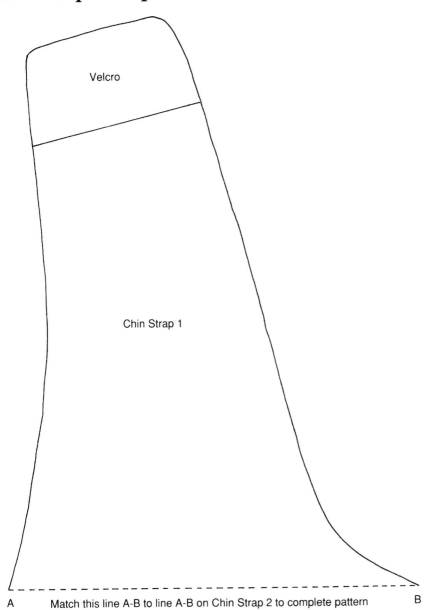

Velcro

Chin Strap 1

A   Match this line A-B to line A-B on Chin Strap 2 to complete pattern   B

Chin strap 2 template

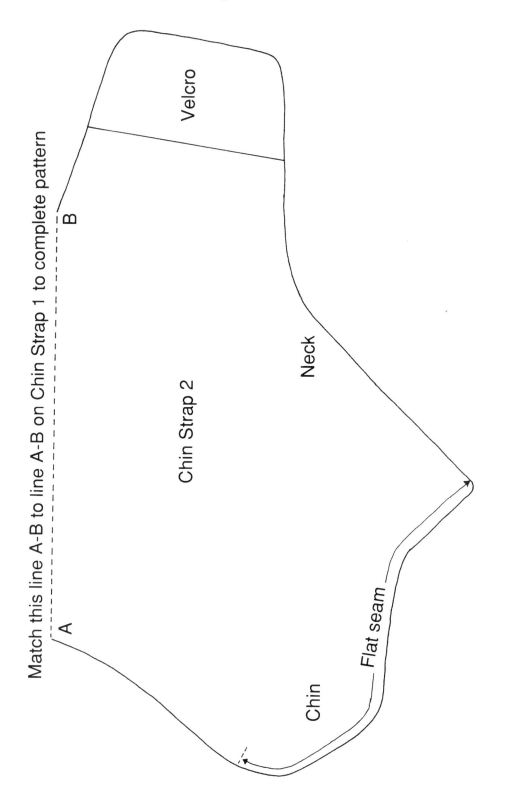

Velcro

B

Match this line A-B to line A-B on Chin Strap 1 to complete pattern

Neck

Chin Strap 2

A

Chin

Flat seam

7

Modified garments

Please read the general directions in Chapter 2 before making any garments. The applications of pressure garments are not limited to treatment of hypertrophic scarring. They are also used for lymph-oedema management, splinting and for oedema control in amputated limbs. The possibilities for these garments have not yet been fully exploited. As you increase your experience and understanding of the use of pressure garments, you will be able to expand the range of their application. In this chapter, we hope to challenge you with one example.

Pressure garments are helpful in reducing stump oedema in the early stages following amputation. They are made for those patients who:

(i) have bulbous or misshapen stumps, and
(ii) cannot be fitted with standard-sized commercially-made garments.

The length of the stump will determine the garment design. Garments for below-knee/elbow or long above-knee/elbow stumps can be secured by having soft elastic sewn into the inside of the top of the sock alone. Shorter above-knee/elbow stumps will need to have extensions which will anchor the garments. These extensions are similar to:

(i) the top of the single legging for lower limb stumps, or
(ii) in the case of above-elbow stumps, the half vest design.

Below-knee stump sock

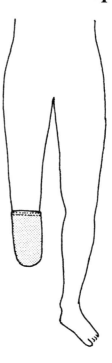

1. Measurements

1a. To make a below-knee stump sock use measuring chart number 4 in Appendix III.

1b. Measure for the length of the stump sock with the knee in extension. Measure from the tip of the stump to the knee joint crease.

1c. Circumferential measurements are taken at 5 cm intervals from the knee joint crease to the widest point at the end of the stump. It is not necessary to measure the end of the stump, as this will be accommodated for later when the garment is fitted.

2. Drafting the pattern

2a. Unlike other sock designs, do not adjust the stump length line as this will occur when the garment is fitted. Adjust the circumferential measurements by multiplying them all by 0.4.

2b. Using a ruler, draw a vertical line on a blank piece of paper to represent the knee–stump tip length. Mark the top end of this line **K**nee and the other **T**ip.

2c. The adjusted circumferential measurements are plotted horizontally so that they are bisected by the vertical length line. This can be achieved by dividing each circumferential measurement by two, to halve them. One half is plotted on each side of the length line with small x's. Ensure that these marks are accurately spaced.

2d. Connect these measurements at the top with a straight line to form the top of the pattern (Figure 7.1).

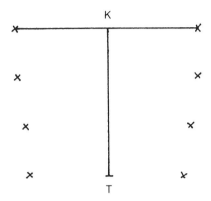

Figure 7.1 **Circumferential marks (K, knee; T, tip of stump)**

2e. Join the x's on each side with a smooth line to approximate the stump contours.

2f. Flare the pattern at the top end by no more than 1.5 cm on either side (Figure 7.2).

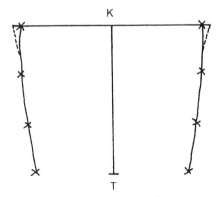

Figure 7.2 **Flared pattern**

2g. Next, draw a horizontal dotted line equal to the width of the pattern, 5 cm distal to the end of the length line. Connect the sides of the pattern to this line with light pencil marks (Figure 7.3). Cut this pattern out carefully.

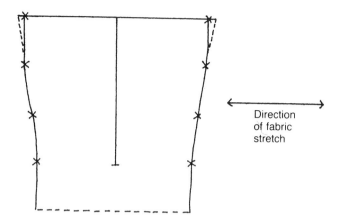

Figure 7.3 **Provisional pattern**

3. Cutting the fabric

3a. Pin the pattern onto a doubled piece of fabric, ensuring that the direction of stretch corresponds with the circumferential calf measurements and not with the length.

3b. Cut the fabric out, following the pattern lines accurately. Remove the pattern.

4. Sewing the garment

4a. With wrong sides together, pin and sew one side seam with a zigzag stitch of 0.5 cm width.

4b. Open the fabric and measure the width of the sock top. Cut a piece of soft elastic (as described in Chapter 2), and sew into place along the inside edge of the sock top, using a long zigzag stitch (Figure 7.4).

4c. Pin and sew together the remaining side seam with a zigzag stitch of 0.5 cm width. *Note*: The distal end of this garment is still left open at this stage.

5. Fitting and completing the garment

5a. Have the patient don the garment. Using one hand to hold the front and the back pieces of the garment together, draw a line around the stump outline directly onto the fabric (Figure 7.5).

5b. Remove garment from the patient. Sew the two pieces of fabric together, following the outline accurately with a 0.5 cm wide zigzag stitch (Figure 7.6).

Elastic

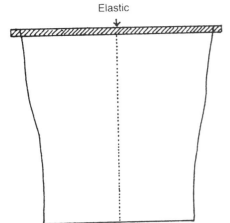

Figure 7.4 **Position of the elastic**

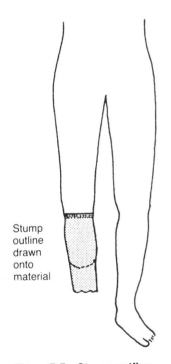

Stump
outline
drawn
onto
material

Figure 7.5 **Stump outline**

5c. Once a satisfactory fit has been achieved, trim away excess fabric
    and mark the final stump outline onto the pattern for future refer-
    ence. This completes the garment (Figure 7.7).

Medial 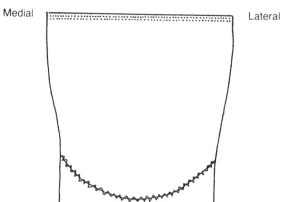 Lateral

Figure 7.6 **The sewn stump outline**

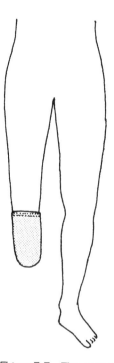

Figure 7.7 **The completed stump sock**

References and useful reading

Artz, C.P., Moncrief, J.A. and Pruitt B.A. (1979) *Burns: A Team Approach*, W. B. Saunders, London

Barnett, P.H. and Stafford, F.S. (1984) Use of plastic air bands for edema and scar contractures. *Journal of Burn Care and Rehabilitation*, **5**(6), 469–473

Baur, P.S., Larson, D.L., Stacey, T.R., Barratt, G.F. and Dobrkovsky, M. (1976) Ultrastructural analysis of pressure-treated human hypertrophic scars. *Journal of Trauma*, **16**(12), 958–967

Cheng, J.C.Y., Evans, J.H., Leung, K.S., Clark, J.A., Choy, T.T.C. and Leung P.C. (1984) Pressure therapy in the treatment of post-burn hypertrophic scar – a critical look into its usefulness and fallacies by pressure monitoring. *Burns*, **10**, 154–163

Clark, R.A.F. and Henson, P.M. (1988) *The Molecular and Cellular Biology of Wound Repair*, 3–23

Cooper, and Prockop, 1968 in Kischer, C.W., Shetlar, M.R. and Shetlar, C.L. (1975) Alteration of hypertrophic scars induced by mechanical pressure. *Arch. Dermatologica*, **111**, 60–64

Covey, M.H. (1988) Application of CPM devices with burn patients. *Journal of Burn Care and Rehabilitation*, **9**(5)

Datubo-Brown, D.D. (1990) Keloids: a review of the literature. *British Journal of Plastic Surgery*, **43**, 70–77

Davey, R.D., Wallis, K.A. and Bowering, K. (1991) Adhesive contact media – an update on graft fixation and burn scar management. *Burns*, **17**(4), 313–319

Deitch, E.A., Wheelan, T.M., Paige Rose, M., Clothier, F. and Cotter, J. (1983) Hypertrophic burn scars: analysis of variables. *Journal of Trauma*, **23**(10)

Fujimore, R., Hiramoto, M. and Ofuji, S. (1968) Sponge fixation method for treatment of early scars. *Plastic and Reconstructive Surgery*, Oct., 322–327

Gallagher, J., Goldfarb, W., Slater, H. and Rogosky-Grassi, R. (1990) Survey of the treatment modalities for the prevention of hypertrophic facial scars. *Journal of Burn Care and Rehabilitation*, **11**(2), 118–120

Gollop, R. (1988) The use of silicone gel sheets in the control of hypertrophic scar tissue. *British Journal of Occupational Therapy*, **51**(7), 248–249

Harries, C.A. and Pegg, S.P. (1989) Measuring pressure under burns garments using the Oxford Pressure Monitor. *Burns*, **15**(3), 187–189

Holmes, J.D., Muir, I.F.K. and Rayner, C.R.W. (1983) A hypothesis of the healing of deep dermal burns and the significance for treatment. *British Journal of Surgery*, **70**, 611–613

Hunt, T.K. (1984) Can repair processes be stimulated by modulators (cell growth factors, angiogenic factors etc.) without adversely affecting normal processes? *Journal of Trauma*, **s39–46**, no. 9, supplement

Johnson, C.L. (1984) Physical therapists as scar modifiers. *Physical Therapy*, **64**(9), 1381–1387

Kischer, C.W., Bunce III, H. and Shetlar, M.R. (1978) Mast cell analysis in hypertrophic scars, hypertrophic scars treated with pressure and mature scars. *Journal of Investigative Dermatology*, **70**, 355–357

Kischer, C.W., Shetlar, M.R. and Shetlar, C.L. (1975) Alteration of hypertrophic scars induced by mechanical pressure. *Arch. Dermatologica*, **111**, 60–64

Kloti, J. and Pochon, J-P. (1979) Long-term therapy of second and third degree burns in children using Jobst-compression suits. *Scandinavian Journal of Plastic Reconstructive Surgery*, **13**, 163–166

Larson, D.L., Abston, S., Evans, E.B., Dobrkovsky, M. and Linares, H.A. (1971) Techniques for decreasing scar formation and contractures in the burned patient. *Journal of Trauma*, **11**(10)

Lawrence, J.C. (1987) The aetiology of scars. *Burns*, **13**, s3–s14

Leung, K.S., Cheng, J.C.Y., Ma, G.F.Y., Clark, J.A. and Leung P.C. (1984) Complications of pressure therapy for post-burn hypertrophic scars. *Burns*, **10**, 434–438

Leung, P.C. and Ng, M. (1980) Pressure treatment for hypertrophic scars resulting from burns. *Burns*, **6**, 244–250

Longacre, J.J., Berry, H.K., Basom, C.R. and Townsend, S.F. (1976) The effects of Z-plasty on hypertrophic scars. *Scandinavian Journal of Plastic Reconstructive Surgery*, **10**, 113–128

McDonald, W.S. and Deitch, E.A. (1987) Hypertrophic skin grafts in burned patients: a prospective analysis of variables. *Journal of Trauma*, **27**(2)

Mallick, M.H. and Carr, J.A. (1982) *Manual on Management of the Burn Patient*, Harmaville Rehabilitation Center, Pittsburg, PA, USA

Nelson, J. (1978) The prevention and treatment of hypertrophic scars using pressure garments. *British Journal of Occupational Therapy*, 158–163

Perkins, K., Bruce Davey, R. and Wallis, K. (1987) Current materials and techniques used in a burn scar management programme. *Burns*, **13**(5), s406–s410

Perkins, K., Davey, R.B. and Wallis, K.A. (1983) Silicone gel: a new treatment for burn scars and contractures. *Burns*, **9**, 201–204

Pratt, B.J. (1992) An investigation into the outcome of pressure therapy on hypertrophic scarring. *MSc thesis* (unpublished), University of Southampton, UK

Robertson, J.C., Hodgson, B., Druett, J.E. and Druett, J. (1980) Pressure therapy for hypertrophic scarring: preliminary communications. *Journal of the Royal Society of Medicine*, **73**, 348–354

Rooks, C. (1982) Pressure vest for babies and toddlers. *British Journal of Occupational Therapy*, 385

Seddon, I.B. and Church, R.E. (1983) *Practical Dermatology*, 4th edn, Edward Arnold, London, 10–14

Spurr, E.D. and Shakespeare, P.G. (1990) Incidence of hypertrophic scarring in burn-injured children. *Burns*, **16**(3), 179–181

Stalheim-Smith, A. and Fitch, G.K. (1993) *Understanding Human Anatomy and Physiology*. West Publishing, MN, USA

Tolhurst, D.E. (1977) Hypertrophic scarring prevented by pressure: a case report. **30**, 218–219

Tortora, G.J. and Grabowski, S.R. (1993) *Principles of Anatomy and Physiology*, 7th edn, Harper Collins, New York

Appendices

I	**Suppliers**
II	**Advice sheet to patients**
III	**Measurement charts**
IV	**Templates: gusset and chin strap**

Appendix I: Suppliers

Lycra fabric: Penn-Nyla Ltd, Acton Road, Long Eaton, Nottingham NG10 1FX, UK (Tel. 0602 734441)

Penn Elastics GMBH, 4790 Paderborn, An Der Talle 20, Germany (Tel. 010 495251 400858)

(Fabric number 25034, but ask for samples to see the range available)

Camp Ltd, Nottingham Road, Long Eaton, Nottingham NG10 1JW, UK (Tel. 0602 732203)

Elastic: Hulme Holberg Ltd, Plants Avenue, Macclesfield, Cheshire SK11 6TP, UK (Tel. 0625 615108)

Thread: English Sewing Ltd, Thread Division, PO Box 12, Stamford Road, Manchester M13 0SL (Ask for F471 Polyfill Cotton, beige)

Zippers: YKK (Fasteners) Ltd, Norwich Avenue, Hunslet, Leeds LS10 2LH, UK

Velcro and Silastic elastomer: Smith and Nephew Medical Ltd, FREEPOST, PO Box 81, Hessle Road, Hull, Humberside HU3 2BR, UK (Tel. 0482 25181)

Silicone gel: Spenco UK Ltd, Burnell Road, Haywards Heath, West Sussex, UK

Talley pressure gauge: Talley Group Ltd, Premier Way, Abbey Park Industrial Estate, Romsey, Hants SO51 9AG, UK (Tel. 0794 830866)

Appendix II: Advice sheet to patients

You will only obtain the maximum benefit from your garment(s) if the following instructions are observed:

1. *Wear* your garments 24 hours a day. Remove them only to wash, massage and cream your scars and to change the garments.
2. *Change* your garments daily.
3. *Avoid* direct sunlight on your scars as this makes them more active. Use a total sun-block cream on them for protection.
4. Your scars may develop a deep red-purple colour as they mature. *Do not worry*, this is quite normal. The colour will fade with time.
5. *Remove* your garment and contact your therapist as soon as possible if any of the following signs occur:

   - swelling
   - 'pins and needles'/prickly sensation
   - blue colour in extremities, e.g. hands, feet, fingertips
   - soreness or breaks in skin.

6. *Do not* cut or alter your garments in any way, as this will disrupt the way they apply pressure to your scars.

Caring for your garments

7. *Hand-wash* in lukewarm water, using a mild soap. Dry at *room temperature* and not on a radiator or in a tumble-drier.
8. *Protect* your garments and skin when doing housework/manual activities by using e.g. gardening gloves, etc., when appropriate.
9. If your garments become worn, slack or damaged they will not work well. Check with your therapist before discarding them.
10. Your garments will need to be *replaced regularly*. On average, gloves are replaced at 6 weeks and other garments by 12 weeks of use. Contact your therapist in advance to have new ones sent to you. Occasionally, you may need to be remeasured to ensure a good fit. An appointment can be made for this purpose. If you have any questions or problems about your pressure therapy, do not hesitate to contact:

    Therapist: _____
    Tel.: _____

Appendix III: Measurement charts

Chart No. 1: Below-elbow sleeve

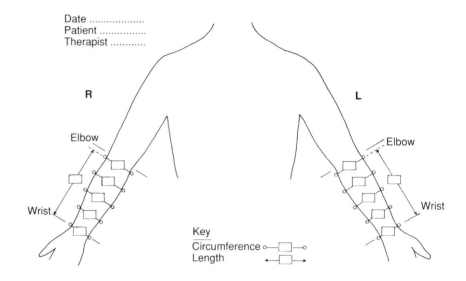

Chart No. 2: Jacket

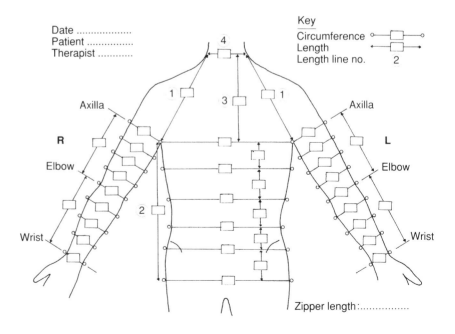

Chart No. 3: Leggings/shorts

Key

Circumference

Length

Date ....
Patient ....
Therapist ....

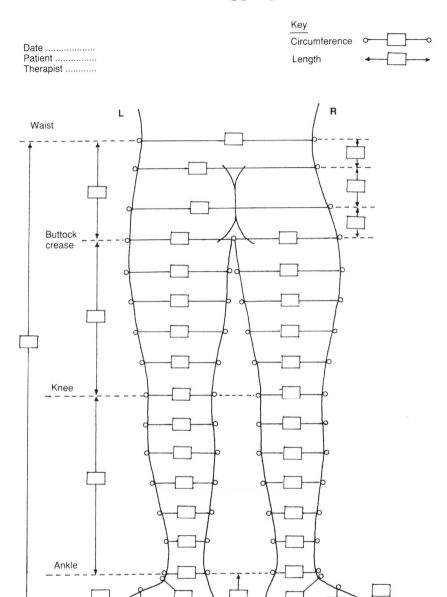

L   R

Waist

Buttock
crease

Knee

Ankle

Chart No. 4: Below-knee sock

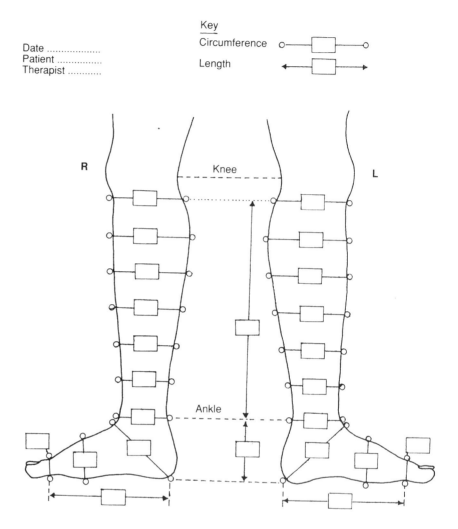

Chart No. 5: Full mask

Key

Circumference

Length

Date ....
Patient ....
Therapist ....

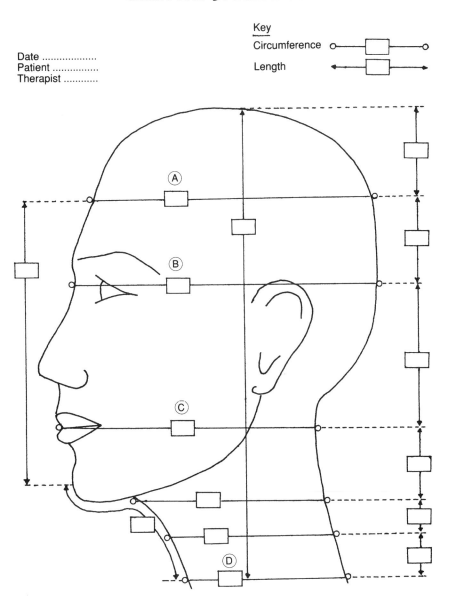

Chart No. 6: Chin strap

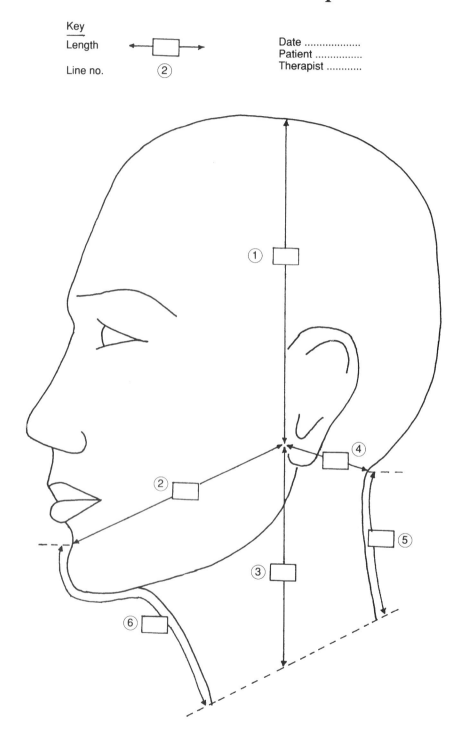

Appendix IV: Templates

Glove gusset template

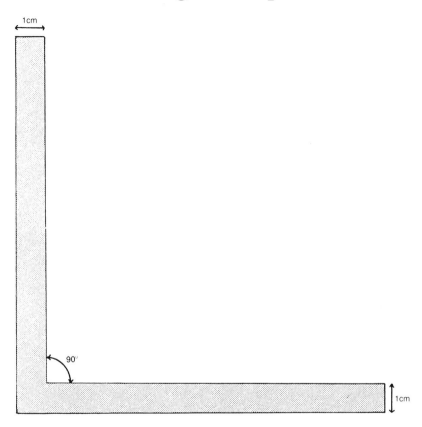

1cm

90°

1cm

Chin strap 1 template

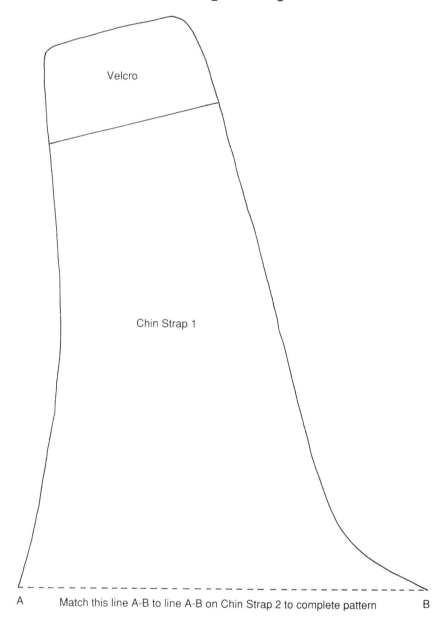

Velcro

Chin Strap 1

A   Match this line A-B to line A-B on Chin Strap 2 to complete pattern   B

Chin strap 2 template

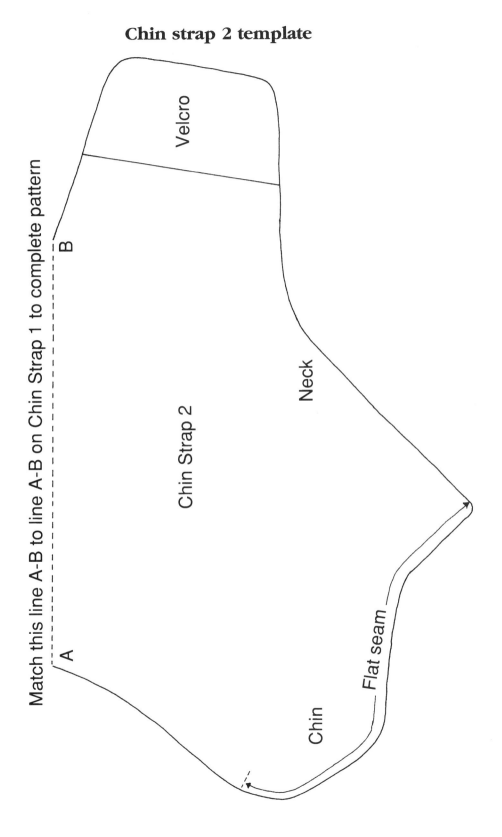

Match this line A-B to line A-B on Chin Strap 1 to complete pattern

B

A

Velcro

Chin Strap 2

Neck

Chin

Flat seam

Index